The End

Of

A Diabetes Journey

Memoirs of a Grateful Man

Dave Livingston

Copyright © 2014   William David Livingston

All rights reserved.

ISBN 10:149592114X

ISBN 13: 978-1495921148

To

Bobby

... you changed my life and never knew it.

Introduction

At the age of twenty-four, my life was forever changed with the diagnosis of type one, juvenile diabetes. I quickly realized that learning all I could about diabetes would offer the best strategy I could take to live as long as possible while avoiding the life-altering complications of this disease, or as I prefer to call diabetes, condition.

I wanted to share my story with those who find themselves searching for someone who has lived with diabetes a long time and can possibly benefit from that person's experiences. It is good to know others have faced this diagnosis and continued to maintain a positive lifestyle while working toward a successful future. I am not an expert in the field of diabetes nor a writer. I do not have any medical certification or training. I am simply a guy with day to day experience. I did not always do the right things to help myself as I should have done. I often felt angry having to deal with this condition, a condition which lies on the mind of the diabetic individual each and every day.

I have taken a look back at my life with diabetes by the decade, from the initial diagnosis until today. Hopefully those diagnosed with diabetes today will benefit greatly from recent advances in treatment and technology that were not available years ago. Type two diabetes has become so prevalent today, and it also has the potential to cause life-changing problems for those dealing with its effects.

Today, I no longer have diabetes, and I wanted to share that miracle as well. By telling my story I hope to bring encouragement to those with diabetes and let them know their futures can be bright. I encourage those with either type one or type two diabetes to take control of their health and realize that today's efforts make a positive difference in their lives years into the future. I would also like to encourage an awareness of the early indicators for type two diabetes in order to prevent it from occurring if at all possible. If I can help just one individual with diabetes live a more enjoyable life by sharing my story, then I have accomplished what I hoped to do.

Chapter 1

A need to thank a friend. . . .

We made the long drive from north Alabama to the historic and serene country graveyard near Savannah, Georgia. I am sure it is difficult for someone to understand my motivation for traveling that distance to visit an individual grave site, but it was a journey I felt compelled to make. After all, I needed this visit to say, "Thank you," to someone I owed so much. It was the least I could do for someone who had done so much to make my life so much better. I simply needed a few moments alone to reflect on what this person had done for me so selflessly. This young man had died so suddenly; a young man whom I had never met, yet I think of each and every day. I had wanted to place flowers on his grave but since there were so many already in place, I didn't think I should add more. I decided instead to write a message expressing my feelings on a card, seal it in a plastic bag and tape it securely to the beautiful stone his family had chosen for him. I wanted to do more, but this was at least something I could do to let his family know how much his gift had meant to me.

Bobby, whom I had come so far to visit, died in a motorcycle crash the previous year. He was an organ donor, and I had received his pancreas and one kidney. I am sure organs were given to others, yet I had no way of knowing, and it really didn't matter. I just felt compelled to let someone know how his gift had affected me. I stood by his grave and thought about the thirty-five years of insulin injections and the other associated problems that I had experienced over the years such as diabetic retinopathy and kidney failure. I needed to make this visit.

When I think back to first hearing the word "diabetic," I can still recall the feeling I had deep inside my stomach. I had never been inside a hospital with the exception of being born, so I always felt I was extremely healthy and never had anything to complain about when it came to illness. I had easily passed each of my navy physicals, and I never felt sick. I never had a headache, earache or toothache during childhood. Other than the usual childhood illnesses, I had been a healthy young guy. I had been told my grandmother had had diabetes, but she had passed away the year I was born, so I never actually knew her. My father had never forgotten how she struggled to take her daily insulin injections as he watched her cry and plead to avoid having to take the shots. That memory stayed with him the remainder of his life.

I had been told that she discovered diabetes after losing part of a toe to this disease. She probably had diabetes for a long time without knowing and lost her toe probably because of her high blood sugar. On my mother's side of the family tree, several cousins had type one diabetes. One cousin had actually been an early kidney transplant recipient. Since his brother was a good donor match, he was able to donate a kidney. The diabetes gene was definitely hiding in my family tree. In the late forties and early fifties during my grandmother's era, diabetes management was primitive compared to what it is today. Large needles, which had to be sharpened, and sterilized glass syringes were used to inject insulin. This image of my grandmother who had to endure this procedure had stayed with me from childhood until the day I was told that I, too, had diabetes. I will always remember the look on my dad's face when I first told him that I also had been given the same diagnosis as my grandmother. He had remembered how my grandmother had dealt with diabetes, and the only words he could say were, "Oh no."

I assured him I would be all right, that medical advancements had been made in the last twenty years or so, from nineteen-fifty to the early seventies. In reality, I had no idea what had changed; I only wanted to reassure him at the time.

When I turned seventeen, I was one of those young boys who joined the Naval Reserve while in high school, and by the time I was twenty-three, I was completing my six-year enlistment. I had also worked my way through college in order to earn a teaching degree, and I had just begun my second year teaching middle school.

I had just begun work on my master's degree, and that meant many trips to the University of Alabama at Birmingham, a ninety minute drive from my home in North Alabama. I noticed that I was often thirsty and would stop to buy a soft drink on the way there. I didn't think much of this at first, but as time went by, I had to stop twice during the drive and also make sure I had something to drink during class. I stayed extremely thirsty.

Since I was adjusting to this routine over a period of time, I didn't realize that something was happening to my body. I did notice I was using the bathroom quite often, but I attributed that to the amount of fluid I was consuming each day. All-in-all, life was good at that moment. I had a great job in a progressive school system, and I was also working toward a master's degree. Life could not have been better. I had worked a job during the four and one-half years I was in college and had not enjoyed a free Saturday or Friday night during that time. I was enjoying a normal workweek routine, and I was extremely grateful for everything that so many people had done to help me reach that point in my life.

People began to ask, "What are you doing to lose weight?" "Nothing," I would reply. "Well, you look good, " would be their follow-up response. I was never really overweight, but getting slim was a nice feeling. It was nice to hear someone compliment me for looking slender.

Before long, the complimentary tone of someone asking what I was doing to lose weight, changed to, "You are losing too much weight; you need to stop." When the annual class pictures were made, I took a hard look at my photo and compared it to the one made the previous year. The image I was seeing let me know something was not right. My eyes seemed to be set in a hollow face, my cheek bones seemed to protrude where I had never seen them before, and I didn't look healthy. I didn't like what I was seeing.

One of my co-workers and I were talking one morning, and she asked if I was dieting in order to lose weight. I told her definitely "No," I did not diet, and ate anything I ever wanted. I told her I stayed extremely thirsty all the time. Her eyes opened wide as she said to me, "You are diabetic." I laughed and told her, "No," that I was not diabetic. I couldn't be, not me." She said to me "Oh yes, you are! I have an aunt who had the same symptoms, and she is diabetic." After I thought about it a minute, maybe she had something to at least consider. But I still wasn't willing to admit that I might have diabetes. I struggled to stay involved with the seventh grade class I taught each day. I had little energy and seemed to stay exhausted. In those days it was a common teaching practice to use a film projector and show some sort of filmstrip during class. I remember being so lethargic that simply turning the projector knob seemed a tiring chore.

I decided that I should find some sort of information to try and learn something about diabetes, so I dropped by a local drugstore and picked up a magazine which had an article devoted to diabetes. I was amazed when I read the information in the article. The author could have easily been writing about ME. No ifs, ands, or buts about it, I had the classic symptoms mentioned in the article: extreme thirst, drinking anything to excess, accompanied by frequent bathroom visits. I didn't realize it then but I was becoming dehydrated. I was losing weight even though I was not dieting.

I made the decision to talk to a doctor, and that was something I was not accustomed to. I had not seen a civilian doctor since I was about five years old when the diagnosis was made that I needed a tonsillectomy, or so claimed the family doctor. My mother and father looked at each other and said we would go home and think about it and get back with him. Without hospital insurance and the money to pay for an operation, they needed an exit strategy to get out of the doctor's office. It seems that in the nineteen-fifties there were a lot of kids who supposedly needed tonsillectomies for some reason. Looking back, I believe it was really more of a fad than a needed surgery. Since we didn't have the money, I never did get the tonsillectomy. I had never needed a doctor since then, but now I needed one. I called a local doctor's office, explained my symptoms and was told I needed a "glucose tolerance test." I didn't really understand what glucose was. I thought it was something they gave accident victims to keep them living or something. I did not know it is actually another name for sugar (or glucose) in the bloodstream.

As I waited in the doctor's outer office to begin the glucose tolerance test, I sat across from an elderly gentleman who was missing one leg. There were only the two of us waiting, so in a short while we began a conversation about the usual things most people have in common- weather, seasonal changes, and such. After awhile, the old gentleman asked me, "What are you here for?"

"A glucose tolerance test," I said. "I think I might have diabetes." The old gentleman slapped the upper portion of his amputated leg and said to me, "That's what happened to my leg." I suddenly felt a sick feeling deep in my stomach.

Within a few minutes I was taken from the waiting room to begin the glucose tolerance test. I would never see the old man again, but I have never forgotten him.

In the seventies a glucose tolerance test took about four hours to complete. A patient drank a bottle of thick sugar solution and during that time several blood samples were drawn and checked by a lab technician to determine the rise in the glucose level as it traveled through the bloodstream. I was sure that I was diabetic, having read additional material and having talked with various people who knew about diabetes and its symptoms.

It was then time to meet with the doctor and learn my test results. When he came in the room he quickly said, "Well, you made a good diagnosis. You are definitely diabetic." I wanted to know more so I asked, "How bad diabetic am I?" "I don't know," he said, "my machine goes up to 400 and yours kept climbing. I can't say how high your blood sugar really is. I would say that you are what I would call a 'walking coma.' "A normal glucose reading would have been around 100. Although the news was not good, it had at least not come as a great surprise. By then I had mentally prepared myself for his diagnosis. He recommended that I begin insulin injections immediately. I asked him, "Can't you give me some sort of pill?" I could not stand the thought of having to take a shot each day, and I would be willing to take any sort of pill if that might be an alternative treatment. He said he didn't think oral medication would work in my case, but he would be willing to prescribe it for me to try. I began taking the pills and my blood sugar showed improvement in a matter of weeks. Checking blood sugar in those days meant a visit to a lab where blood was drawn from a vein, sent to a lab and results returned after several days. I took the pills for the next two years and watched what I ate as best I could. I asked the doctor for advice about what to eat. He said, "don't eat bread, sweets, and potatoes." That was the diet advice given in the early seventies by a family doctor. I tried to drink the only sugar free soda available in those days, a soft drink called "Tab." I could not drink it then, and I cannot drink it even today. Learning to cook was something I never had the patience to do, and even today I am not one of those men who enjoys standing in the back yard over a barbecue grill with a spatula in one hand and a fork in the other as they grill something.

    I searched to find a doctor who could offer more information about diabetes so I chose a specialist in internal medicine. He gave me detailed information about the diabetic diet, and I began to understand the importance of trying to balance my food intake with the right amount of protein, fats, and carbohydrates. I learned that foods could be grouped in categories based upon their characteristics. This was called the "Exchange Plan." I then had to know the approximate number of servings allowed at each meal to meet my dietary needs.

    I learned to cook "bachelor style," so I had time at night to work on school papers and projects to get ready for the next day's lessons. Only teachers know what this is all about. Most people leave work and go home to relax, most teachers leave work to go home and work some more. I discovered a counter top broiler oven was a much better cooking device than a full size oven especially when broiling a small piece of meat such as a four-ounce portion of ham or beef. I could pop the meat in the broiler oven, and in a few minutes it was cooked. Clean up was easy, too. I could open a can of green beans and heat them with some instant potatoes and a slice of toast, and there it was, a meal fit for a king. Well, it was filling anyway. Breakfast was easy since it could be a combination of individual parts. One egg, one or two pieces of bacon, one or two pieces of toast, or one-half cup of low-sugar cereal, and similar breakfast items could easily be calculated in the exchange diet depending on the meal plan with the prescribed number of total calories. I did try to follow my meal planning and calorie counting within reason. No one is usually perfect all the time when it comes to eating what they should, and I wasn't either. I avoided the items heavy in sugar such as syrup, jams, jellies, and soft drinks. In the early seventies there were very few sugar-free products which tasted good to me. Today, there are a number of products available which are made with improved sugar-free sweeteners and actually taste quite good. Many of these are made using natural sweeteners, too. I would suggest to anyone today to seek out a dietician with the latest information about what is currently available. I feel any affordable product which makes life with diabetes easier is a good thing.

    I learned to keep my eating plan pretty well under control when I was at home. It was the time away from home that usually caused me trouble. My mother was the traditional southern cook. If it wasn't fried in Snowdrift shortening, it wasn't up to her standards. She would almost seem insulted when I ate a normal amount of food. To her, food and love went together. If you didn't want at least one extra helping of something, that meant you didn't enjoy it. More than once I tried to explain to her why I needed to eat right, but I don't think she ever really understood. And, of course, she always had homemade desserts which were so difficult to say "no thanks" to, as she insisted I eat at least some. Whenever I made a visit, I was supposed to eat and then eat some more.

    School related functions where food was spread before me on tables was often a challenge to avoid as well. I learned to pick one or two small items with less sugar and hold them on a paper napkin or paper plate as I talked with people. I found that kept them from asking why I wasn't eating something. To me, managing what I ate was just as important as taking my medication. I began to look at my health and keeping blood sugar under control. I had to be aware of three very important components to stay healthy:

1. Oral medication or insulin

    I always took my medication as prescribed. During my first two years with diabetes, I relied on oral medication to help control my blood sugar. Taking insulin meant new changes to adapt to once again. I will explain more about insulin later. I have heard some people simply decide at some time to skip their medication or insulin injections because it is inconvenient. When I left home at four in the morning to go on a long drive to fish, I would prepare my insulin dosage, and, just before stopping to eat breakfast, I would give myself an injection. I have heard that some people who crave sweets actually take extra insulin before eating desserts. I never did that and don't think it is a good thing to do.

2. Food

    It is just as important for someone on insulin to eat, as it is to avoid eating. The food is needed in order for the insulin to have something to metabolize into energy. I learned through years of experience that getting in a low blood sugar situation was something I wanted to avoid if at all possible. On a couple of occasions I found myself at the hospital emergency room being given glucose intravenously in order to bring me back to consciousness. Over a period of years I developed a sensitivity to insulin, or insulin resistance. My blood sugar would often drop suddenly, and I had to find something sweet to eat quickly. I also learned that any amount of alcohol could cause my blood sugar to drop suddenly since my body was working to process the alcohol rather than deal with the insulin and blood sugar. This could happen with only one lite beer, so I drank only an occasional lite beer and tried to be aware of what might happen.

Eating too much food at one time can cause the blood sugar to elevate, especially if too many carbohydrates are consumed. I tried to use common sense when it came to eating.

3. Exercise

I learned over the years that I felt much better staying active and not sitting in front of the television so much. I liked to be on the move at school, especially after I became a school principal, moving from room to room during the day and interacting with the staff and students. For many years I have been a member of a fitness facility, and I go there to exercise regularly. I don't have to go there to exercise, I could exercise at home, but I enjoy the company of other people, and it has become a part of my daily routine. After I exercised, I felt more energetic, and my blood sugar stayed under much better control. This didn't mean I was a muscle-bound weight lifter or marathon runner, I was certainly none of those, but I tried to work some sort of regular exercise into my daily activities. This might be a lot of vigorous walking, brisk walking on a treadmill, swimming, or any other activity that made me burn extra calories.

If it sounds as if having diabetes requires learning to balance medication, food and exercise in order to be as healthy as possible, then that is true. This is a daily routine which many people cannot seem to discipline themselves to follow. Those who do, however; seem to avoid many of the problems associated with diabetes over a longer period of time than those who don't. I noticed over time that I was hardly absent from work due to illness. I believe staying active and eating healthily helped me avoid many other illnesses.

Chapter 2

The importance of knowing. . . .

    Although I became adjusted to the idea that I was someone with diabetes, I had a lot to learn in order to live normally. I was single, so cooking and meal planning was not something I enjoyed doing. It is difficult today to imagine a time not so long ago without computers and the internet where we can easily locate and gather information about diabetes or any other subject. In my early days with diabetes I searched and found magazines and sources which gave me information about foods to eat and foods to avoid, recommended types of exercise, and other topics which might help me. I also found a doctor knowledgeable in the area of diabetes, an "internist." In this case the term "internist" refers to a doctor specializing in internal medicine, not a "doctor in training." I felt an internist had more training in diabetes than other doctors and would probably keep more abreast of the latest available information. I made three individual appointments with separate doctors before choosing the one I thought would help me most. I wanted someone I could communicate with, rather than someone who would be all-knowing and simply a dispenser of information and medicine. I wanted a doctor with whom I could work as a partner in my treatment. I needed someone who could be a good listener.

    Shortly before becoming diabetic I met a girl and we briefly dated. At that time I mentioned to her that I thought I might be diabetic and would be having some tests done to determine if it were true. We were not at a point that we would be getting serious, so for several months we dated other people. We later started dating seriously, and I told her that I had been diagnosed with diabetes. I enjoyed being with her, but I wanted her to know about my diagnosis. She didn't seem to mind. I was taking part in any activity anyone else might be doing, I was only trying to watch my food intake, staying away from the "bread, sweets, and potatoes" I had been earlier told to do, and of course taking my oral medication, my pills. Life was about to take a major change however.

After dating several months we decided to get married. I almost felt guilty asking her to marry me since I had heard stories about the terrible effects diabetes can have on someone, I also remembered the old gentleman with the amputated leg. I had kept that image in my mind. Maybe that has been a good thing, I'm not sure. Just before we were married, I learned the local health department offered classes on diabetes, so I signed up to attend. I also mentioned that, if we were going to be married, she might as well go and learn along with me. We both went to the classes which met once each week, and we both learned together. We learned as a team. We learned about food groups and how food impacts blood sugar levels as it is broken down in the body. We learned about the grouping of foods in what was called an "exchange group," meaning that a serving of food in one group was equivalent to a portion of another food from that same food group. I could understand that a single piece of loaf bread had about the same amount of carbohydrates, fat, calories, etc. as one-half cup of creamed potatoes. I just had to know the number of servings I could have from each "exchange group." It made a lot of sense to me, and I learned first that breakfast was an easy meal to plan as was lunch since I carried a sandwich, apple, or other fruit and maybe a small bag of chips and unsweetened tea. The night meal was something similar the way it was planned, only it was more involved with vegetables, meats, etc. It meant I could have a variety of vegetables, meats, even bread and potatoes. I just had to watch portion size and not eat way too much. I could live with that. We didn't have the money to eat out very much anyway, and we learned that a small hamburger, diet drink and small fry were okay. It didn't mean a half pound hamburger and large fries were however. My wife, Alice, adapted to cooking with little frying in oil, and we each learned that eating "diabetic food" is nothing more than eating "good food." Since she has been cooking this way for more than thirty-seven years, she has gotten very good at preparing some tasty and healthy meals. Since our son never had lots of junk food around home while growing up, he never became hooked on them and learned to eat healthier food as well. As one doctor told me years ago, everyone should be eating a diabetic diet.

In the classes, I learned a lot of important things about diabetes, things I had never even thought about earlier. I had really never thought much about what diabetes is in the first place. I thought it was just something that happens to someone, when, in reality, it is the inability of the body to process glucose or blood sugar properly so we can use it for energy. I learned there are two basic types of diabetes. Type one, usually called juvenile diabetes often shows up in many very young people. It can even happen to infants. The general thought about type one diabetes is that it is caused by some sort of genetic condition. Over the years I heard theories that it might be caused by everything from someone having unprocessed cows' milk as a child, to lack of vitamin D, toxins in the air, and other theories that I can't even remember. This form of diabetes is characterized by a very fast change in metabolism which seems to indicate that something happens suddenly to kill the insulin producing cells. I seemed to fit this pattern for sure. I was told quite early that I was, in fact, a type one or juvenile diabetic. To this day, I do not think there is any clear understanding as to why some people become a type one diabetic. I don't think it is anything God has put upon us. I don't think we bring it upon ourselves. I think it just happens. Whatever the reason, the insulin producing cells attached no longer function causing the blood sugar to rise. Unless this insulin is replaced through injections, the patient will eventually die and face a host of complications beforehand.

What a joke! Twenty-four years old and a type one, juvenile diabetic! At that time I didn't realize some very public personalities also had type one, juvenile diabetes. The actresses, Mary Tyler Moore and Halle Berry are two well-known people who have done quite well in spite of their type one diabetes. Brett Michaels and Nick Jonas, rock music stars, are also type one diabetics. Those people who have type one diabetes require insulin since their pancreas produces little or no insulin at all.

The other form of diabetes we hear so much about today is called type two. Often this condition is caused by the body's inability to produce enough insulin, or the insulin produced is not working just right for some reason. Many times when someone has gotten older and gained a lot of extra weight, their body cannot produce enough insulin due to larger body mass. That, coupled with a lack of exercise, causes a rise in blood sugar. Doctors can often prescribe oral medication to make the pancreas produce additional insulin. The oral medication combined with diet and exercise can help many people. Types one and two cover the vast majority of people.

An easy way to remember the difference between type one and type two is to think of this:

Type two diabetes without medication causes sickness; most often, good control can be achieved through diet, exercise, and perhaps medication. According to the National Diabetes Education Program, type two diabetes accounts for 90 to 95 percent of diagnosed cases of diabetes in adults.

Type one diabetes requires insulin, or diabetes will lead to death. That's a very simple way to think about the difference, but that pretty-well sums it up. I fit in the type one category, even though I was able to get by for a short time taking the oral medication. Approximately 5 percent of adults with diabetes are type one.

Gestational diabetes occurs in two to 10 percent of pregnancies. Women who have had gestational diabetes have a 35 to 60 percent chances of developing diabetes, mostly type two, in the next 10 to 20 years.

My pancreas was producing some insulin years ago, and the oral medication simply pushed my pancreas to work harder. It helped me to process the insulin I was producing. I'm not really sure how, but I was at least getting by. I still did not feel good, and the smell of certain foods cooking often caused me to feel nauseous. I had little appetite. I was trying to do the best I could to cope with this new lifestyle.

One night during the diabetes class our lesson was about insulin and the injecting of insulin . . . the dreaded "shot." When our instructor, Marcie, announced that we would be learning how to do an injection, I asked her privately if I could give myself an injection rather than use the skin of the orange she had provided. She seemed puzzled as to why I would want to do this, and I explained that I only wanted to see if I could actually stick my self with the needle, I suppose to see if I were man enough to do this. She thought about it a few seconds and said that it would be fine, she would let me do this in front of the class.

I wasn't certain if I really wanted to give myself an injection in front of the class; I thought I could, but I hated to have spectators. Now that I remember years later, some of those people looked as nervous as I was then. Marcie laid the items out on the table in front of the room as others looked on. There were a small plastic wrapped injection syringe, an alcohol swab, and a bottle of sterilized water to use. She opened the package containing the disposable syringe and the pad with the alcohol and swabbed the rubber top to the bottle of sterile water. Finally, she asked, "Where do you want to give yourself the shot?"

"In my stomach," I told her.

"Why in your stomach?" she asked.

" I believe if I can give myself a shot there, then I can do it anywhere," I said. After instructing me to use the alcohol swab and clean a spot on my stomach, she handed me the syringe, and I promptly inserted the needle and emptied the sterile water into my lower abdomen. She commented that I would not have a problem giving myself an injection, and I never did. I later knew a man who stayed in the hospital an extra five days, because he could not be released until he gave himself an injection.

It really was an easy process. The glass syringe I had remembered hearing my father mention from my grandmother's era had been replaced by a small plastic syringe with a very small needle. The needle was so small I hardly felt anything when it went through the skin. I was still very happy to not have this routine to follow each day. *We* learned so much valuable information from those classes. I realized then that I could give myself insulin injections if I had to. I didn't want to, but I could. Some people have a fear of needles, but I did not have to overcome that obstacle.

Marcie taught us about the importance of insulin or prescribed medicines. She showed how to choose a variety of foods and taught us about the food exchange groups. She emphasized the importance of proper foot care, and why poor blood sugar control often leads to amputations and organ damage. She stressed the importance of regular vision checkups since diabetes can damage the tiny blood vessels of the eye and so many other things which I could never have picked up simply by reading. Knowledge about diabetes is a good thing. I don't really consider diabetes my enemy, but I don't consider it my friend either. Regardless, I wanted to know all I could about this new game I would be playing for the rest of my life. I made a decision early on that diabetes was the hand of cards I had been dealt. I intended to play to win.

For several months I was able to maintain some sort of blood sugar control by using the oral medication. Although I didn't feel great, I had avoided insulin since I still resisted the daily routine of taking injections. When I went to the doctor and had my blood sugar checked, the result would usually be considered high by today's standards, but back then it was okay. My doctor said if I could keep it less than 180, I would be fine. That number is not considered fine today for sure.

A normal blood glucose range today is generally thought of as near 100. I believe in the seventies it was thought of as anything below 120 for someone who did not have diabetes. Mine was staying around 150 if I remember correctly today, a number which would not be good by today's standards with improved technology.

I continued to take the oral medication, the pills, until my doctor told me this particular medication had been removed from the market since it possibly caused heart related problems in some patients. He said there were a couple of others we could try, but he was not optimistic because the one I was using had been his best choice for me, and the others had not shown good results. After trying both of those medications, my blood sugar showed up extremely high on each lab report causing my doctor to deliver some news I had dreaded so much hearing. I needed to be put on insulin. Although I had given myself that injection during diabetic class, I still didn't want to get in this routine each day, but it seemed I had no choice. He said he would schedule the hospital for a few days so I could be monitored for the proper amount of insulin and determine how I would react. I could feel that sick feeling deep down in my stomach once again.

Once in the hospital, I began the process of giving myself the insulin injections. During the day and night my blood was drawn and tested to see what my blood sugar levels were running. I was instructed to be up and walking around the hospital during the day, and I was *not* to stay in bed. That seemed odd, I was in the hospital walking around, going all over the place in my street clothes as sick people watched me walk past their rooms. Friends visiting the hospital would ask me who I was there to see, and I would tell them, "No one. I am in the hospital." That explanation usually brought a laugh, and I would further explain why I was there and what the doctor had told me to do. I was only following doctor orders. He wanted to adjust my insulin level to match my usual daily routine as closely as possible.

The one thing I began to notice was that I had more energy than I had known for a very long time. I soon realized that I had cheated myself by not wanting to try insulin months earlier. My body was working better on the insulin injections. I noticed the nausea often experienced from the oral medication was gone also. Food seemed to smell better, too. I soon felt better and had more energy to work with the kids at school. The fear of the dreaded insulin shots had kept me from getting my best medicine. It was time to move forward.

Chapter 3

New technology changes things . . .

Just as changes had been made from the early nineteen-fifties, when my grandmother had to cope with sharpening needles in order to re-use them, changes today and new advancements are continually making life better for the person with diabetes.

The disposable syringe with the tiny attached needle used today was a tremendous advancement for those in the past who had to sterilize syringes and sharpen needles in order to take insulin. That also meant more portability and easier travel for the diabetic patient too, something we now take for granted.

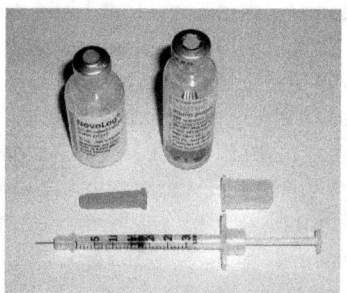

Bottles of a lifesaving insulin and modern disposable syringe.
Courtesy of National Institute of Health

In the seventies, blood testing meant a trip to the lab where blood was drawn from a large vein using a big needle and then sent to a lab for testing. Thanks to the home blood glucose monitors available today, checking blood sugar is easy to do and with little pain. I remember the first home blood sugar monitor I ever saw. It was probably in the mid-eighties. I recall an ad in some sort of diabetic magazine illustrating a new device which would allow an individual to check their blood glucose level at home. I thought, "This is just what I need," and promptly ordered one. Upon receiving it, I opened the package and began reading the instructions to use the device. It has been so long ago that I can only vaguely remember them today, but I recall there were several steps which had to be followed in a proper sequence to complete a successful test. The kit included a plastic wash bottle, finger pricks, alcohol swabs, color test strips and color chart which were all laid out before use. The test also required a time keeping device which had a second hand in order to monitor the precise time needed for each step. Once the finger was pricked, blood was quickly applied to the test strip and allowed to dry for a specified time, then the wash bottle was used to rinse the blood spot for a specified number of seconds, then a second rinse after so long, and so forth. Then the test strip color was compared to a color chart on the meter which gave some sort of number range indicating the amount of sugar floating around in the bloodstream. I found the process so cumbersome that I soon quit using the device completely. But this was a first step in the development of the blood glucose monitors in use today. I was so excited when I found the early meter that I took it to my doctor who had no idea something like it existed. I even tried to demonstrate it to him but since the process took so much time, I gave him an overview instead and left before completing the blood test. But once again, it was a start toward a better means of treatment. Today, there are so many glucose monitors available that choosing the one best suited to the patient's needs is the hardest decision to make. Just as cell phones have become more reliable and able to perform so many functions, technology has also improved glucose monitors making them very reliable and affordable. There are new models which can actually measure the blood glucose without the need to draw a blood sample. There are dozens of glucose monitors available from which to choose. When I became diabetic, the only method to measure glucose at home was a type of litmus paper which was passed through the urine stream. The paper would change color based upon the amount of sugar in the urine. I had trouble even doing this since I am basically color blind. I could not differentiate the color variation so I needed Alice to help me compare the colors. The results were inaccurate anyway, but it was the best tool available at that time. As I mentioned earlier, there are so many dietary related items available today that were not available in the seventies to make life easier with diabetes and more enjoyable. At that time, saccharin was the only artificial sweetener on the market. Honey, a natural sweetener, is not usually recommended for diabetic use since it is still sugar and can raise blood sugar levels if too much is consumed. Occasionally I rewarded myself with honey as a treat, rather than as a staple of my diet.

Today, I do not drink soft drinks of any kind and I will explain why later, but in the seventies I hated not being able to drink regular soft drinks such as Coca-Cola, Dr. Pepper or Pepsi. They each had too much sugar. I later enjoyed diet Pepsi when it became available. The sugar substitute, Splenda, became the sweetener I liked better than some of the others, although today there are those who claim it is not a healthy alternative to sugar due to its unnatural origin. Being diabetic often requires making choices, I chose to use Splenda in moderation as I learned to do in a lot of things. Moderation is probably good to always keep in mind. There are a number of other sugar-free products that would take too long to list. I really like some of the sugar free ice cream products which taste good in my opinion. If I didn't know before tasting them, I would say they were made with sugar. Once again, just because it lists sugar free on the package does not mean I can eat as much as I want, it still contains calories of some sort, and all food turns to glucose. Some foods just turn more quickly than others.

Today, we often hear someone ask a fellow friend with diabetes, "What was your A1c this time?" They were referring to the A1c test or score, which is a number correlating to the long term blood sugar level. This number is important since it lets the patient know how well blood sugar is controlled over a period of weeks rather than what the blood sugar might have been on one particular day. This is so important to know since a good A1c number relates to good control which lessens the chances of complications such as nerve damage, possible blindness and amputations. These tragedies can occur over time when elevated blood sugar levels are left unchecked. Maintaining a good blood sugar number should be the goal of all people with diabetes. Maintaining good control today helps prevent problems in the future.

With the development of laser technology, treatments for diabetic retinopathy are now available. The retina, located in the back of the eye is damaged when excess blood sugar causes new blood vessels to grow on the retina. These blood vessels grow on the retina, slough off and eventually lead to blindness if left untreated. The laser is used to send a strong beam of intense light which breaks up these rogue blood vessels before the retina is completely covered. Blindness from diabetes today is uncommon due to advanced treatment, but blindness can happen.

In my earlier years, checking blood sugar required a visit to a lab to have blood drawn by a technician or nurse. Years later when glucose monitors became available for home monitoring, I was lax when it came to checking my blood sugar on a regular basis. The early glucose monitors required a drop of blood from a fingertip, and even today I hate to have my fingers pricked. Finger tips are really a sensitive part of the body to stick with a sharp instrument. Today's glucose monitors allow blood to be taken from a small area on the arm where there are very few nerve endings. I became much more diligent about monitoring my blood sugar when these monitors became available.

Many people with diabetes have found great success with the insulin pump available today. I learned over a long period of time to keep my blood sugar regulated through multiple injections. Due to that reason I did not ever try an insulin pump. Although pumps are great for many people, each person must decide what is best for him or her. One thing I have really enjoyed many years is water recreation. I felt the pump would be difficult to use during the summer months when I enjoyed being in the lake. My doctor and I discussed the issue of trying a pump but I chose instead to continue with injections. My A1c number was always good so there did not seem to be a reason to change. There may be pumps available today which could have successfully worked for me, but I don't really know.

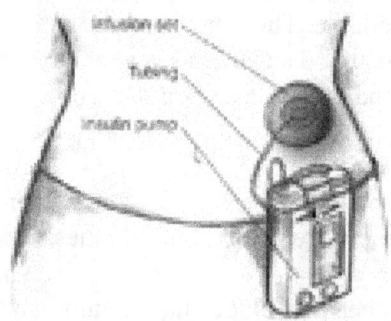

Insulin pump illustration
Courtesy of National Institute of Health

Newer forms of insulin have been developed and help to maintain better blood sugar control than was available several years ago. In the past insulin was derived from cattle or hogs and contained impurities which sometimes led to injection site sensitivity or other problems. Insulin marketed today is created and grown in a laboratory and offers a variety of options to meet the patient's individual needs. It is quite routine for an individual to use a mixture of insulin each day to provide a better level of control than years earlier. It is so important that someone with diabetes work with a doctor familiar with the latest products available. This field of medicine and associated technology is constantly changing and continually being updated.

1.
The name "diabetes" is attributed to the famed Greek physician Aretaeus of Cappadocia who practiced in the first century A.D. He believed diabetes was caused by snakebite.

Chapter 4

During my twenties . . .

From my twentieth birthday to my thirtieth, I experienced a lot of things, some really good things and a few not so good. As I mentioned earlier, I was about twenty-four when I became diabetic, seemingly from nowhere with no known cause. I learned all I could about diabetes, and I was determined to not be like the old gentleman with the amputated leg I had met at the first doctor's office.

My wife and I were married when I was twenty-seven, and, in a year or so, we began the process of building a new house. Before we married she often mentioned how she really liked log style homes, so we soon bought a few acres and made plans to build one. We wanted to do a lot of the work ourselves, but we knew we would need someone to do the bulk of the major construction. Any work we could do, we did ourselves in order to save money. The men worked during the day and we worked after our regular work day. We also worked each weekend until the house was finished. We had to move into our home before it was completely finished since we had sold our other home and needed to move. We did not want to move twice, so we were roughing it for a while in the new location.

One night I wanted to finish installing some work upstairs, so I worked until midnight, installing flooring, causing me to burn a lot of calories. I was so exhausted when finished that I went straight to bed and fell asleep from sheer exhaustion. The next morning Alice came in and had trouble waking me. She attributed this to the night before since I had worked so hard, so late. She finally brought me a scrambled egg, bacon and some toast and gently made me sit up to eat, assuming I was groggy from lack of sleep. I do not remember anything to this day about that breakfast. Standing in front of the kitchen sink with my head spinning as I stared into the distance was the first thing I can recall. My head was pounding from an excruciating headache. As she saw me standing there, appearing as if in a trance, she began to ask questions, some of which I had trouble answering.

I could not imagine what was happening to me, but finally, I could start to see my surroundings more clearly. In a few minutes I went back to bed since I did not feel like working. I did not know what had happened, but I had actually experienced my first INSULIN REACTION. I had used so much physical energy, so much blood sugar, that my blood sugar had dropped during my sleep, and I did not know it. Had I eaten something more just before bed I probably would not have experienced the low blood sugar episode, or at least not that badly anyway. I had not realized the correlation between insulin, food, and exercise until then. It was a hard lesson to learn.

When I'm watching television, I often notice mistakes made about diabetes. They use the term diabetic coma a lot. I guess that sounds a lot more dramatic than "insulin reaction." An insulin reaction is brought on by LOW blood sugar. A diabetic coma is the result of extremely HIGH blood sugar. Neither condition is good, and both should be avoided. I have seen someone portrayed as diabetic and non respondent. Inevitably, someone says that the individual needs insulin. If that person has passed out due to low blood sugar, the shot of insulin in a real-life situation would drive the victim's blood sugar even lower. It could even cause death. More than likely that person needed a piece of candy instead. I learned to carry something sweet with me in case I began to show the signs of low blood sugar. I found the little individually wrapped pieces of peanut butter candy to be my candy of choice. They are easy to open and easily eaten when needed if I wanted to get the sugar in my system quickly. They dissolve quickly when hard candy can sometimes take too long. A sugared soft drink can provide the sugar needed but I always wanted something in my pocket for immediate use, locating a coke might not always be easy to do. My lips would begin to tingle when I began to experience low blood sugar. I would sometimes stare into space as if concentrating on something, when in fact I was not thinking about anything in particular. My heart would beat much faster, too. Probably the greatest indicator was the feeling that I needed something sweet to eat right at that moment. Some of those indicators changed as I became older and my body adjusted to insulin.

Years later I would experience low blood sugar more quickly, perhaps due to my efforts to keep my blood sugar from going too high. Keeping blood sugar within range can be a true balancing act at times.

In my twenties I had no other health related problems. My eyesight was fine, checkups were always good. In those days there was no A1c number to be of concern. When I had my blood sugar checked about every three months, I was told it was fine. There wasn't much else I could do anyway to make it better, so I continued with my daily injection, ate about the same things from day to day and did about anything anyone else did for fun. I didn't eat a lot of the things people my age usually enjoyed, and I stayed away from too much pizza and the jumbo-sized fast food orders.

Our son was born when I was thirty. I worried that he might inherit the diabetes gene, but years later he has no sign of diabetes. Since he grew up in a home with little candy, sweets, pastries and junk food, he learned to eat a lot of the healthier foods. When my twenties came to an end, I was teaching fourth grade, we had built a home, we had a new son and life was good. I had adjusted to being a person with diabetes. I sometimes resent being called a "diabetic" even though I throw the word around frequently also. Calling some one a diabetic is describing what that person does, a carpenter, a plumber, a doctor. I did not "do" diabetes. Since the world has become very politically sensitive about anything and everything today, I don't take issue with being called "a diabetic." I realize it is a convenient term to use. There are more important things in the world to worry over.

My twenties' decade was a time of change for me, and also a great time, too. I went from being single, to husband and father. I became a teacher in a great school system, and I also finished my enlistment in the Naval Reserve. Later in my twenties I completed my Master's degree and did post masters work as well. Soon after turning thirty years old I became the principal of a school which served kids with special needs. I accomplished most of this while dealing with diabetes. I wanted to control the diabetes; I didn't want it to control me. At the end of my twenties I was so grateful for the good life I was enjoying.

2.
Ancient doctors would test for diabetes by tasting the urine of a suspected sufferer of diabetes. Sweet urine is high in glucose suggesting the presence of diabetes.

Chapter 5

Diabetes is a really big deal . . .

When we look at someone who is dealing with diabetes, he or she does not usually exhibit any outward signs of being someone with a health problem, yet this image is deceptive. Uncontrolled diabetes means the person's blood sugar is much too high for a long period of time. This extra blood sugar surging through the blood stream is damaging the tiny blood vessels in vital organs such as the eyes and kidneys. If left uncontrolled, this high blood sugar can lead to blindness, kidney failure, heart disease and other problems. These conditions are life-changing and should be avoided if at all possible. Many people who have diabetes think it can never happen to them, so they don't take their condition seriously. Vision loss and kidney damage can occur even when the person worked diligently to maintain a stable blood sugar and practiced good control. No matter how good the oral medication or insulin we take is, it is still not the same as the insulin our pancreas makes. I wanted to at least postpone those problems until old age if I possibly could. The longer I kept my diabetes under good control, the later in life I hoped it would be before I experienced eye or kidney related problems.

One serious problem related to the eyes is diabetic retinopathy. As explained to me by my retina specialist, the retina is a part of the eye which can actually send out tiny blood vessels as it searches for oxygen it is lacking due to excess blood sugar in minute blood vessels. These tiny blood vessels grow over a period of time and actually act much like tree roots growing on the ground near a tree as they cover the retina. They eventually die causing changes in vision leading to blindness if left untreated. A thorough eye exam is strongly recommended for someone with diabetes, even though there may not be any outward signs of vision change. Diabetes does its damage silently. It is like a thief in the night which can bring surprises if left unattended. I was about twenty years old when my vision was checked in the Navy, and I was told I needed to have a second look at the eye chart. I asked the corpsman, "Why do I need to repeat the eye chart?"

"Because you did too good," he said. I had shown in one eye 20/10 and 20/15 in the other. This was a much better score than the standard 20/20.

At about thirty years old I had another eye exam, and the doctor finished the exam by saying he did not see any signs of diabetes damage, and commented, "Son, you have the eyes of an eagle." That made me feel good, I was always concerned about my vision and wanted to take good care of my eyes. In my later thirties, I as most people, needed reading glasses and I accepted that as just part of the aging process. When I was in my early forties, I decided it was time for another eye exam since it had been several years since the last one, and I made an appointment with a new doctor. My first doctor had retired. After the doctor finished the exam, he gave me some news I was not expecting to hear. He said, "you have diabetic retinopathy." I will explain in more detail about laser surgery later.

Keeping blood sugar under good control can help prevent or at least postpone many of the problems uncontrolled diabetes can cause. What is done today to maintain better blood sugar control helps prevent problems in the future.

Diabetes can take a toll on the kidneys also. The kidneys are vulnerable to the high blood pressure that usually accompanies diabetes. Even though I had tried to keep my blood sugar under good control, I had been living with type one diabetes for thirty-five years. During my fifties I learned from my regular doctor that I was beginning to show signs of kidney damage, and that sometime in the near future I would require dialysis. This news came as a shock, but I could still enjoy those things I wanted. I enjoyed my boat, swimming, and having fun during the summer. I lived with this diagnosis for ten years until it finally came true.

People who have diabetes have the potential to develop circulatory problems. The old gentleman I first mentioned with the leg amputation, I am sure, was an example of this. He dealt with diabetes before the development of the personal blood glucose monitors and his blood sugar may have stayed elevated for long periods of time. This caused a lack of blood circulation to his feet and lower legs. People who have diabetes also need to closely examine their feet for any signs of infection, or cuts which if left untreated can cause serious problems.

One habit I never acquired was smoking. When I was young, I bought an occasional pack of cigarettes but I never really enjoyed smoking them. I am happy that I did not develop the habit. One reason I suppose I didn't was due to cost. I never felt I had the money to buy them anyway. Years later I enjoyed cigars while in my boat fishing, but I never inhaled the smoke as most cigar smokers seem to enjoy the relaxation that a cigar brings. I later quit buying them also when I decided that I was wasting money and I could better utilize my time paying more attention to my fishing rather than fumbling around with cigars.

I would recommend that anyone who smokes and has diabetes stop smoking as soon as possible. There is just too much information available which supports the fact that cigarette smoking is particularly detrimental to the person with diabetes. I have recently read a study suggesting that nicotine bonds with blood sugar to actually make the A1C, or long term blood sugar, level rise. The study discouraged the use of nicotine patches since they also release nicotine into the bloodstream. The only real option for a smoker with diabetes is to stop smoking completely. I am sure this is very difficult for a heavy smoker to do, but it is at least something important to consider.

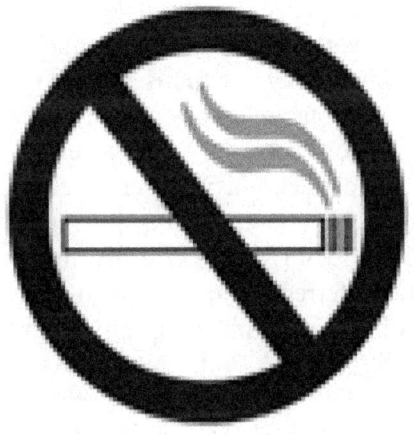

Courtesy of National Institute of Health
National Institute of Diabetes
Digestive and Kidney Diseases

Chapter 6

My thirties . . .

I would call my thirties a time of "maintaining." I had learned in my twenties to deal with the daily routine of eating consistently. I had not learned many of the things about better nutrition that I know today, but I did stay away from foods containing a lot of sugar. I always followed my regimen and never skipped my injections. During my thirties I discovered that I required more than one injection each day in order to keep my blood sugar under better control. I took one injection early in the morning before breakfast and a second injection just before eating my evening meal. Occasionally I would experience an insulin reaction, and I learned to always carry something with sugar. I learned the little peanut butter log candies were what I preferred. I tried the glucose tablets available at drug stores, but, since I didn't really like carrying a large packet, I stayed with my peanut butter logs.

I walked constantly at school each day, but I felt this was probably not as much exercise as I needed. I joined an exercise facility and went there each afternoon after school to add more workouts to my routine. I did some weight training and swam in order to get some aerobic exercise. I liked the feeling exercise gave me, and it seemed to make me feel better mentally. Being responsible for a school and all the things that take place there is a stressful situation, and stress has a direct impact on blood sugar and overall health. I found that doing some good aerobic exercise at the end of the work day helped me to alleviate the day's stress. I seemed to sleep better also. I enjoyed having some place to go after work before going home. I tried to leave a lot of the day's problems there. I didn't get to leave them all, but at least it did help. The exercise also gave me the feeling that I was in control of my health to a large degree. I felt good most of the time. I sometimes heard people complain about not feeling well, yet they had no apparent health problems. I think they really needed to move more. We purchased a lake lot during my thirties, so I found myself each weekend spending a lot of time swimming and water skiing. I have always enjoyed being around water. Having diabetes did not keep me from doing just about anything I wanted to do. We had built a home earlier and did a lot of the work ourselves. We were now working to build a get-away place on the lake that we could enjoy. This meant building a dock and boat house, construction which required a lot of hard physical work. When my blood sugar got low, I ate something to bring it back up. I could tell from the shaky and nervous feeling I would get when it began to drop. My lips would also tingle. This was an early warning sign I could recognize. Other people might have signs they know as low blood sugar warning signals, but those were my signs. I also needed to have something with real sugar available when I was out in the boat far from the dock. After water skiing for a long while I would find I needed something to eat just as if I had been working extremely hard. I learned that physical exercise helped to keep my blood sugar lower.

It seems hard to believe today with all the available blood glucose monitors on the market, but it was during my thirties that they became so common and readily available. What a change this made for so many people! No longer did it require a doctor's visit in order to get a blood sugar reading. It could be done quickly and easily anywhere, at any time. The latest monitors allowed the blood to be withdrawn from a place on the fatty part of the lower arm. This was a great improvement, since few nerve endings are located there, so the process was virtually painless. I began to check my blood sugar a lot more often when I did not have to prick my fingertips.

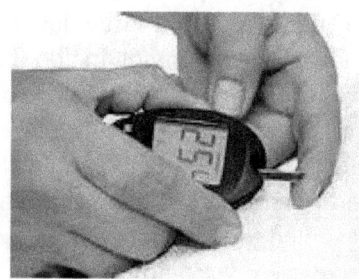

Courtesy of
National Institute of Diabetes
Digestive and Kidney Diseases
National Institute of Health

During my late thirties I began to notice a rise in my blood pressure. I did not realize the relationship that blood pressure and blood sugar share. The excess sugar floating around within blood vessels causes inflammation, which has the effect of elevating blood pressure. Sometimes blood pressure changes with age for some people, and mine was beginning to show the effects of nearly twenty years of diabetes. Although I had tried to follow all the rules and be consistent with my diabetes management, I could not maintain insulin levels as consistently as a properly functioning pancreas.

The decade of my thirties was a great time for me. I had been through the stress of a major school renovation, my school Parent Teacher Association had achieved 100% membership and the community seemed to be so proud of the new building's modern renovation. We enjoyed our weekends at our lake home, and my overall health was good. Each day I carried a lunch from home which usually consisted of a peanut butter and banana or cheese sandwich, a small bag of chips and fruit, usually an apple. Sometimes I either brought a diet drink for lunch or drank unsweetened tea in the school cafeteria. I avoided the school lunches due to the amount of fat and carbohydrates they usually contained. School lunches are prepared for active, growing school kids. They are not necessarily good for adults, and certainly not good for people with diabetes in most cases.

One time of day that often gave me trouble was the time directly after school, from about three until four o'clock. My lunch was usually around noon, and, by that time of day, my blood sugar would often tend to get low. I would need to eat something in order to avoid an insulin reaction. That time after school was also the time when a parent might drop by upset over something related to school that day. I needed to be able to deal with people and problems each afternoon at that time. I learned to prepare and eat a snack as soon as possible after the last bell rang in case I might experience low blood sugar. I remember one particular experience when an upset parent was sitting in front of me as my blood sugar kept dropping. At that moment I felt I could not ask the parent to wait while I popped a couple of peanut butter bars into my mouth to bring my blood glucose up to a normal range. I survived that particular situation, but I did not want it to happen again. The same scenario could also happen in large meetings where I could not easily leave to find something sweet to treat low blood sugar.

I always had plenty of sugary peanut butter candies in my pocket for those kinds of events. Many people prefer peppermint candies or something similar. It doesn't really matter as long as it is something made with real sugar and not a sugar substitute.

The decade of my thirties was also the decade of the eighties. When I think back to the seventies, I realize major advancements were made during the eighties which improved the lives of those living with diabetes, especially those with type one, juvenile diabetes. The development of new types of insulin and improved testing methods helped many people obtain better control than had ever been possible in the past. Insulin pumps were developed during that time period, and many people found them to be great tools to obtain better blood sugar control. Regardless of the method of testing used, the insulin prescribed, or the type of insulin delivery, it is still up to the patient to use diligence each and every day in order to keep blood sugar under good control. With good diabetes management, there is never a holiday. There is never a vacation from being in charge. Those who decide to ignore their insulin or overeat during the holiday season usually get in trouble and sometimes even require a hospital visit to get back in control. Being a good diabetic patient requires a great deal of self-discipline. Some people have more self-discipline than others.

I believe I was fortunate to have developed some good self-discipline before diabetes came along. I had learned self-discipline from working during high school and also working to put myself through college while fulfilling my commitment with the Naval Reserve. I had learned early in life that each action we take has a result, some good and some not so good. At least I realized the seriousness of diabetes and I did not want to experience the negative side effects if at all possible.

Chapter 7

All good food is not always good for you . . .

Those first words from the doctor telling me to avoid "bread, sweets and potatoes," were the first words of advice I remember ever getting when it came to knowing what to eat, or to avoid eating. I knew back in the seventies that soft drinks contained a large amount of sugar as well as donuts, candy, pies, etc., so I naturally avoided them. I had not yet realized the important role food plays in the overall health of someone with diabetes.

I was instructed to eat a certain number of portions at each meal from several food categories in order to make a combination of fats, proteins, and carbohydrates in the proper ratios, to try and maintain good blood sugar control. The concern with that approach was that it did not consider the fact that many people, particularly children have certain foods they do not want to eat, and some foods they may even avoid. As I have recently read, a new method of insulin therapy has been developed which is based upon the amount and type of food actually eaten. As soon as the meal is finished, the individual calculates the number of calories and carbohydrates consumed and injects a corresponding amount of insulin to match the amount of food eaten. This seems to be a more natural method to achieve better blood sugar control.

Each night as I watch television, I am constantly amazed at the number of advertisements that are geared toward the sale of fast food. In the United

States today, type two diabetes is near epidemic numbers and many health professionals attribute this in part to two factors. (1) high fat, and high calorie packaged foods, (2) large sized fast food items. During the sixties, soft drinks were sold in six ounce bottles; however, when the cola companies tried to outsell the other, each tried to offer the largest size and cheapest price, leading to cola wars.

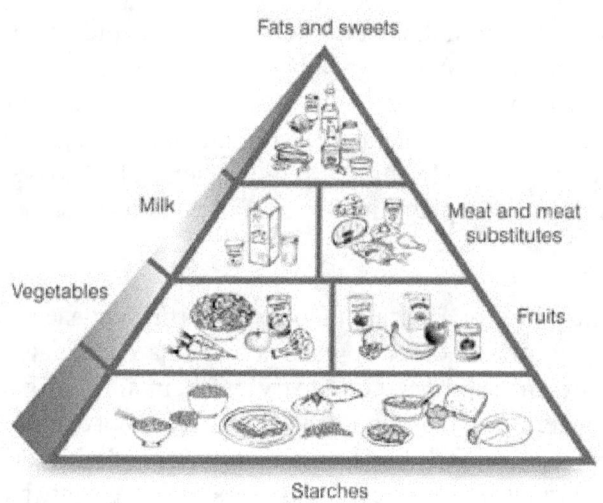

Courtesy of National Diabetes Clearinghouse

The large soft drinks sold today contain little to no food value, and add plenty of empty calories. When we look around and see obese young people, even obese children in elementary school, it is easy to see why there is a rise in type two diabetes. The lack of physical exercise in today's society is another factor I believe is also leading to this rise in type two diabetes. Since we sit in front of the television or spend time on computers we do not move and get the physical exercise we did generations ago. No one seems to walk anywhere, even to the mailbox. Children, who in earlier times would have been out riding bicycles or playing after school, today stay indoors playing video games, missing the physical exercise they once would have gotten. Many health professionals attribute this rise in type two diabetes in children to the rise in childhood obesity.

I have heard people joke about having type two diabetes, evidently thinking diabetes is not serious unless it is type one. Type two can cause the same sort of problem as type one if left untreated. There is nothing funny about either of these conditions.

As so many others who grew up in the south, I was raised on fried food and the extra calories brought about by frying. I had quite an adjustment when I became diabetic and had to develop a new attitude about grilled, broiled or baked food. I am so accustomed to eating food cooked like this today that I have no desire for fried foods. That is amazing to me since I was raised eating fried chicken, fried vegetables, or anything else that could be fried. I never grew up eating salads of any kind, so those were some new food items as well. I enjoy a good salad today, especially with a small amount of good olive oil and vinegar dressing. I have grown very fond of one particular brand, "Newman's Own," which is sponsored by the late actor Paul Newman's foundation with proceeds going to charity. I like good salads too, those that are made with the dark green lettuce and red and green peppers and other good fresh vegetables. It really defeats the reason for eating a healthy salad when it is mostly croutons, potato salad, and heavy dressing poured on top of iceberg lettuce. Many people do not know that iceberg lettuce has little or no food value, but to restaurants, it is cheap and easier to prepare, and it sells. Extra calories lead to additional weight and extra weight means a larger body mass. Type two diabetes can often be attributed to excess weight. Those who have type one diabetes and require insulin need to maintain a reasonable body weight in order to keep the insulin level stable. When an overweight individual loses even a small amount of weight, type two diabetes symptoms can actually disappear. Losing weight often means a change to less insulin for the type one diabetic.

Another benefit from maintaining a desirable weight is the amount of new energy someone enjoys after the weight loss. Another way to be realistic about one's weight is to determine the Body Mass Index. A common internet search for Body Mass Index, or "BMI," will lead to this information which indicates the ratio of height to weight. The resultant score is used to identify underweight, normal weight, overweight and obese. This is an important piece of information which anyone can use to help determine desired weight. The BMI is something to consider and perhaps discuss with a health professional before any changes to medication or even diet plans are considered. It can be shocking when someone calculates their BMI and learns they are in the overweight, or obese category when they thought they were normal weight.

In years past I drank diet soft drinks, especially after becoming diabetic, when I could no longer drink the sweetened soft drinks. I was never an addict, but I did enjoy an occasional soft drink, usually with a hamburger. In my early diabetic days, as I earlier mentioned, a soft drink called TAB was the only soft drink available with an artificial sweetener, and some people seemed to enjoy them. I could never learn to drink TAB. Years later, the Pepsi company came out with Diet Pepsi, and I did like the taste of that product. I enjoyed an occasional Diet Pepsi for many years, but today I do not drink them either. I will explain my reason later.

Eating in restaurants presents another challenge for those who struggle with diabetes management and want to maintain good control. Most of us enjoy the socialization which comes with eating out with friends and family. There are some good restaurant menus geared toward healthier, eating but those tend to be the exception, rather than the rule. Most chain restaurants will serve the food which sells, not necessarily what is good for someone, particularly the person with diabetes. Many menu items contain too many calories, sugar and salt. Before I go to a chain restaurant, I go online and check the menu before I leave home. I check to find the most appropriate item I can order, and also how it can be prepared. Knowing this information before ordering allows me to place my order quickly, saving the server's time. If available, I always order a salad, particularly if one is prepared with Romaine lettuce and better ingredients. I try to plan my meal to total around 500 calories which I can usually do by knowing what I am going to eat beforehand. In this way I get to enjoy other people's company, and still leave the restaurant feeling good about what I ate. I do not go to the places which offer food bars, the "all you can eat" type of buffet restaurant. I don't eat enough to pay for those who do, and, secondly, I don't like places where the customers fill their own plates. That is just my personal preference, since I don't enjoy handling the same serving ladles that others have handled during the day. I just don't feel buffets can be kept sanitary with so many people serving themselves.

    I would also strongly suggest that anyone who is newly diagnosed as diabetic or has been diabetic many years, meet with a certified dietician in order to obtain the latest information available about the foods they should eat. A dietician can also help develop an appropriate meal plan for the individual based upon weight and caloric needs. There are various magazines available which provide great recipes and ideas to make the life of someone with diabetes better. The American Diabetes Association is a great source of information and the organization's magazine, *Diabetes Forecast,* provides recipes geared to the needs of persons with diabetes. Many local health departments offer classes about meal planning and may also provide suggestions for dishes designed to fit the diabetic's eating plan. I never considered myself having to eat a "diabetic diet." I ate just about anything anybody else did; I just learned to eat the right amounts of food according to "my plan." My basic food plan included, vegetables, meats, and fruit, especially fresh fruit. I limited bread and tried to avoid processed meats due to the amount of salt. My lunch each day included an apple, which I learned to consider a healthy dessert. If fresh fruit was not available, I ate unsweetened fruit packed in water to avoid the added sugar of sweetened fruit. I used skim milk when I ate low-sugar breakfast cereal. My overall goal was to limit calories and try to keep my weight down and blood sugar under good control. I was not always successful, but I tried. I dealt with diabetes for thirty-five years.

> 1.
> A Harvard study showed that eating one serving of cooked oatmeal 2 to 4 times a week was linked to a 16% reduction in the risk of developing type 2 diabetes. One serving 5 or 6 times each week was linked to a 39% reduction in risk.

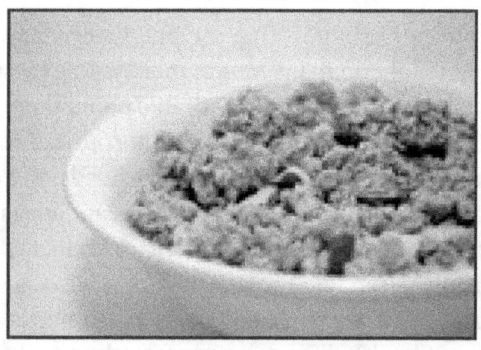

Chapter 8

My forties . . .

When my fortieth birthday came around, I had been managing diabetes for about seventeen years. During this time period the years of diabetes began to show its effects. I had to make lifestyle changes.

I was having trouble keeping my blood sugar within the normal range with two daily injections so I suggested to my doctor that I might need to change my insulin dosage to include a additional injection each day. I had become so accustomed to taking an injection after all those years that additional injections each day didn't seem to be an inconvenience. I found that taking fewer units of insulin several times each day seemed to provide better control. I gave myself as many as five injections as I got older. Besides, if it meant my glucose level would remain normal, then it would be worth doing. I had learned to mix a long-acting insulin with a regular, shorter acting insulin, which seemed to keep my blood sugar under better control. Each weekend at the lake meant skiing, tubing, and having a great time. I could do just about anything any other middle-aged person could, so I didn't feel restricted in any way. My lifestyle was simply adjusted to include daily insulin injections, exercise, and an eating plan which worked to help keep my blood sugar under control. One thing I did not realize at that time was that I was becoming more insulin resistant, meaning my body had become more resistant to the insulin injections over such a long period of time. I found that taking two injections each day did not control my blood sugar as well as one daily injection had done years earlier.

My doctor informed me in my early forties that I was beginning to exhibit signs of kidney damage. I had read that kidney damage can result from long term diabetes, so I didn't panic at the news. He was concerned that my blood pressure was becoming elevated and prescribed medication to help control it. I didn't know that long term diabetes and high blood pressure work together to damage the kidneys. Inflamation caused by blood sugar tends to raise blood pressure, and the high blood pressure weakens the tiny blood vessels in the kidneys helping to further raise the blood pressure. Working together, they create a vicious cycle. Our kidneys are vital to our well-being since they act as filters by removing waste materials in our blood. Although not very big in actual size, they do so much to keep us healthy.

In my late forties I suddenly had to face the prospect of needing kidney dialysis when my doctor informed me that my kidney function was showing a decline with each lab check. I asked how long he thought it might be before I could expect to need dialysis, and he said, "Probably four or five years." Since we each had accumulated nearly thirty years with our retirement systems, my wife and I made the decision to retire early and do some of the things we would not have been able to do should I require dialysis. I had read about dialysis, and I knew that it would be a restrictive lifestyle limiting many of the things we enjoyed. One thing I enjoyed so much was the lake during summer. Even at that age I still enjoyed the water. I hated to think I would lose that important part of my life.

It was during my forties that I developed diabetic retinopathy. Since I had been dealing with diabetes more than twenty years, I suppose time was catching up with me. I was so fortunate to be living during a technological age when lasers could help to preserve my sight. Although the procedure is called laser surgery, there is actually no scalpel or cutting done. A laser is used to remove the tiny blood vessels in the back portion of the eye, the retina. These tiny blood vessels grow on the surface of the retina and affect vision, possibly causing blindness. When I mentioned to a friend that I was probably needing laser surgery, he informed me that he had laser eye surgery a year earlier and was doing quite well. He said the worst part of the procedure was the shot to deaden the eye. I did not have a problem with the small needles used to give insulin injections, but the thought of a long needle near my eye was an entirely different matter. He went on to explain where the needle was inserted and I felt my stomach muscles begin tightening. I have never felt comfortable even putting drops in my eyes, and the thought of a needle so near my eye made me nauseous. I had trouble sleeping several nights as I thought about how I would get through that part of the procedure.

After a thorough examination by a retina specialist, I waited anxiously to hear what she had to say. I suspected the news would not be good. This lady seemed to have a great bedside manner and took extra time explaining how the retina and other parts of the eye work. She explained that the eye is actually much like a camera in a way I could understand. She agreed with the opinion of another doctor that I definitely needed the laser surgery in order to halt progression of the retinopathy. I understood and asked if she would be the doctor to perform the procedure, she said, "Yes," and began to provide more details about the steps she would take and what I would experience. After she finished sharing information with me, I explained to her that I had actually lost sleep just thinking about a needle being inserted anywhere near an eye. She said everyone who goes through this procedure usually had similar feelings. As a matter of fact, she said she usually lost sleep thinking about this part of the surgery also. I told her I thought I could get through the procedure if I could just close my eye and not see the needle coming toward it. She said that would not be possible, since she had to keep my eye completely open in order to make sure there were no problems as she injected the anesthesia. I decided there was nothing more I could do and agreed to the surgery. She asked when I wanted to schedule the procedure, and I told her, "As soon as you possibly can." I did not want to spend time dreading the procedure and losing more sleep than absolutely necessary. I was surprised when she said that she had time available that afternoon, if I would like to begin, and I quickly agreed. She informed one of her assistants that she would be assisting her, and I was taken to another room close by and asked to lie on my back. The assistant stood over me and held my hands to my chest. The doctor then asked me to look to the side and focus on her assistant as she approached from the opposite side with the injection. Since the assistant was a pretty blonde, I joked that keeping my eyes on her would not be a problem. I was told to lie perfectly still as the needle was inserted just to the outer edge of my left eyeball, the needle passing between the eyeball and my cheekbone. I could feel the socket around my eye filling with the fluid from the syringe. She cautiously emptied the syringe and slowly withdrew the needle. I kept my eye closed and waited for the anesthesia to take effect.

When told to open my eye, I could only see darkness. She then escorted me to an adjacent room where I sat in front of a specialized device as she continued to explain about what she would be doing with the laser and what I could expect to feel as she applied more drops to further deaden the eye. She said I would see an extremely bright flash of light, although I could see nothing at that moment. I could not imagine how this machine could focus a beam of light through the lens of my eye to destroy tiny blood vessels in the back of the eye on the retina without damaging other parts of the eye as it passed through, but I was sure she knew exactly what she was doing.

I would hear a loud click each time she fired the laser, and I would then see a flash as if looking directly into the sun. Although my eye had been deadened, I felt a sharp pain each time the laser fired. At the end of the session, she said she had fired the laser about five hundred times. I had a small amount of residual pain, but that was controlled with Tylenol. This was my first session on this eye, and I required another within a few days. Later, the same procedure was performed twice on the other eye. I was grateful this technology existed and happy I had my eyes checked when I did. I had probably saved my vision from further damage, perhaps even losing my vision entirely. My eyesight was not the 20/10, 20/15 it was years earlier, but I was thankful I could see pretty well with glasses. Most people my age had to rely on some kind of eyeglasses anyway, so it didn't seem to matter much to me. I let the faculty know the reason for my black eye at our next faculty meeting. I knew they were curious.

Once again I felt extremely grateful for the knowledge, training, and skill of this doctor. Her expertise and years of training had helped me to keep my eyesight.

> 3.
> Approximately 90% of people with type two diabetes are obese.

Chapter 9

The big 50 . . .

When the doctor told me in my late forties that I could expect to need kidney dialysis within the very next few years, I felt as though life was suddenly coming to an end. I didn't know much about dialysis, but I knew it would bring major changes to my life. I had enjoyed my weekends on the lake, and I assumed that would change also. We made the decision to retire as early as possible in order to travel and enjoy the things we would not be able to do when I had to begin dialysis. Once retired, we bought a travel trailer and began to visit places we had never been before. We visited the Grand Canyon with friends and stayed at our lake home when not on the road in our travel trailer. The four or five-year forecast the doctor had given me about dialysis actually turned out to be ten years.

We were at our lake cabin over a July fourth holiday and had friends down for the weekend. I swam, rode water toys and enjoyed a nice fun-filled weekend. When we came back to our real home, there was a message on our answering machine from my doctor. I had gone in for a lab check before the fourth of July, and he was calling to tell me I needed to report to the hospital as soon as possible. I immediately called his office to speak to him and get more information. He said my kidney function had dropped to the point I would have to begin dialysis. After a great weekend, the news came as a big shock. I tried to convince him to postpone the hospital visit but to no avail. According to him, I had no choice.

I laid the phone down and told Alice the news, which I think she also expected. We began to gather the items I would need while in the hospital and left home, heading directly to the hospital. I had no idea what would be happening when I got there.

My kidney doctor (nephrologist) came in after I was admitted and talked with me about what would be happening during the next few days. The fun-filled past weekend at the lake in the outdoors enjoying the clean, clear water had now changed to that of a hospital environment with the sounds and smells one would find there. I worked hard fighting depression trying to not be a burden to my wife and not exhibit depression to others who came around to visit. In some way I was angry; I just couldn't decide at whom I should direct my anger. I had played according to the rules, but, in my view, I had lost the fight anyway. I wondered why I had been dealt these problems in the first place. I felt I had been cheated. I expressed these feelings to my doctor telling him I felt as if I had failed. He asked, "What do you mean by that?" I told him I never thought dialysis would be something that would happen to me since I had followed the rules, tried to eat and exercise as I should, etc. He then asked, "How long have you been diabetic?" "Thirty-five years," I told him. He then informed that the average patient with diabetes is normally able to live about twenty-five years before needing dialysis. I had made it thirty-five years, ten years longer than average. He complimented me by letting me know that, due to the efforts I had made, I had avoided dialysis ten years longer than the statistical average. That made me feel better, but I still felt cheated by life.

The first order of business was to have an access port inserted in my upper chest which allowed the hospital staff to connect the dialysis machine to my blood supply. This surgery was done as soon as possible and within a day or two I was ready for my first dialysis treatment in the hospital dialysis unit. I was apprehensive, but I assured myself that everyone knew what they were doing, I didn't have a choice anyway. I had unknowingly accumulated a lot of fluid that my kidneys were unable to filter properly, and the dialysis machine was needed to do that. A dialysis procedure lasted about four hours, and during that time I was unable to get up from the chair to move around. Since I don't usually like to sit for very long, I found the last hour extremely hard to endure. This port surgically inserted in my upper chest was actually a tube which had to be protected from the possibility of infection. At the end of that week I was allowed to go home with instructions to begin dialysis at the local dialysis clinic on a regular schedule.

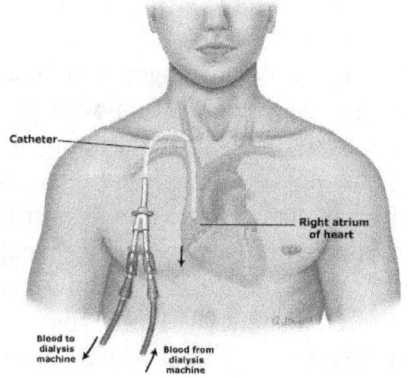

Access port to begin hemo-dialysis
Courtesy National Institute of Health

Life had taken a new turn, but I accepted this change and decided I would make the best of this situation. Others were dealing with dialysis. Some people I knew had done so for years; I could also.

I did not realize how my diet would change when I began dialysis. I had grown accustomed to eating food people with diabetes are taught to eat, but dialysis required a whole new way of thinking. A basic diabetic food plan, or diet, usually considers recommended portions of carbohydrates, fats, and proteins to meet the needs of the individual. Dialysis required that changes be made to the diabetes diet. For years I had been allowed to eat all the garden salads and fresh vegetables I wanted, but dialysis even required that I monitor those, particularly the very healthy dark green variety. These had excess potassium and made dialysis more difficult. As the information pointed out, "too much potassium can cause the heart to stop." I was smart enough to understand that statement. Other foods were not allowed since they could raise my "phosphate" level. That word "phosphate" is a word I heard repeatedly. It seemed just about anything I enjoyed eating contained too much phosphate. Phosphate is difficult to remove through dialysis and can cause bone loss in addition to the extra dialysis time.

   I definitely did not want extra time beyond the required four hours, three times each week, and I certainly did not want to add bone disease to my other problems. Almost all breads of any kind contain a lot of phosphate, so they were pretty well off limits. I was given information about a type of homemade biscuit which could be made using plain flour with no salt and little baking powder. My wife tried this several times but it did not seem worth the trouble to make. The end result reminded me of the hard tack soldiers carried with them during the civil war. Potatoes contain a lot of phosphate, so they were also restricted. I was told to not eat baked potatoes at all. Green vegetables can elevate the potassium level, so they were allowed in strict moderation. The diet sodas I had become accustomed to drinking, since I could not have sugared drinks due to the diabetes, were not allowed as they contain a lot of phosphate and salt. The salt causes fluid retention, and that makes the dialysis process more difficult also. Since I was still dealing with diabetes, I continued to avoid sweets. Those dialysis patients who do not have diabetes are allowed to eat sweets. I was not. The foods I was allowed to eat were corn, since it is very low in phosphate, iceberg lettuce, cabbage, rice, and noodles to name a few, and basically those vegetables which I considered not very healthy. Milk products, such as milk, cheese, and cottage cheese contain a lot of phosphate, so they were strictly limited. I was allowed to have four ounces of milk, or one ounce of cheese each day. The amount of fluid I drank had to be measured since each time I went for dialysis I would be weighed before and after the dialysis treatment to determine how much fluid had been drawn from my body. I thought the diabetic diet had been restrictive, but it was uncomplicated compared to the dialysis diet. Meat, and protein were allowed but in moderation. My daily limit was a total of ten ounces. Alice made major changes to the way she cooked and prepared meals as best she could to help me try and adjust to this new life. Her frustration grew each time she visited the grocery trying to decide just what she could buy to meet my dietary needs. There was so much new information to absorb in a short time period. We were given an instruction manual which outlined specific foods to eat and those to avoid. Liquids had to be carefully monitored. Even sugar-free Jello had to be factored into the daily liquid volume since it is really just a liquid in another form. Ice cream products had to be considered for the amount of phosphate they contain and also the volume of liquid they produce. Many people assume that it is difficult to live and follow a diabetic diet. That cannot be compared to the diet dialysis patients must follow in order to stay as healthy as possible.

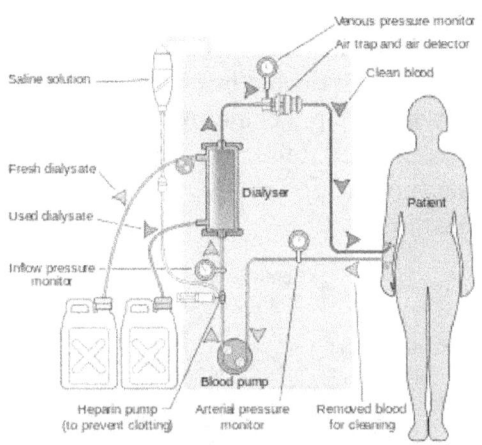

Hemo-dialysis illustration
Courtesy Wiki-commons

My first visit to the local dialysis center was uneventful; the staff was very understanding and extremely patient with me as I began the procedure. The nurse used the port in my chest to attach the tube coming from the dialysis machine, and soon my blood was flowing through the tube, into the machine and back into my body. The room was ringed with chairs and patients who were undergoing dialysis also.

There were people of varying ages and backgrounds not all requiring dialysis due to kidney failure from diabetes. Some had lost their kidneys due to kidney disease or other reasons. The worst part of the process for me was sitting in the chair for the entire four hours. A trip to the bathroom meant the nurse had to disconnect the patient's machine, and start the process again when the patient returned. Televisions were located overhead but since I couldn't find much on television to enjoy, I didn't watch television very much. I did bring my laptop computer, and I saved my morning edition daily online newspaper to read during dialysis. I built a small folding lap table which I could bring with me to support my laptop rather than have it rest on my lap. I could fold it and place it in my carry bag when dialysis was finished. I used my laptop computer to pass the time and make the four-hour period pass by more quickly. The last hour always seemed to pass slowly.

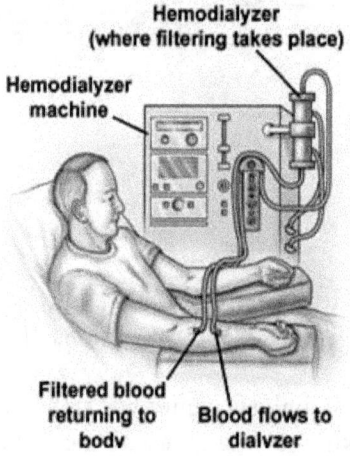

CourtesyWiki-commons

One day during dialysis I heard an elderly gentleman ask one of the nurses to disconnect him from his dialysis machine. He still had a lot of time remaining, and she told him that he was not finished with his dialysis. He said to her, "I don't care, my back is hurting so bad, I can't sit here any longer." Reluctantly the nurse disconnected the man from the machine, and he went to the outer waiting area to await his transportation. I overheard the nurse tell another staff member, "He is being noncompliant." That really bothered me to hear her say that.

I was sure she was frustrated, but I could relate to the way the man was feeling. He was a lot older than I, and had problems staying seated for such a long time. He had age-related back problems, and that only compounded his misery. Not getting the necessary amount of dialysis time would cause him perhaps an extra visit very soon, and it might make him sicker, but, at that point, I don't think he cared any longer. I waited until an appropriate time and asked the lead nurse if she was ever required to sit in a dialysis chair for four hours as part of her training. She said, "No, but that might be a good idea." I agreed with her that I thought it definitely could help those who work with dialysis patients have a little more empathy for those who endure the procedure. I did not mention why I had asked her this question. I grew to have so much respect for the staff who worked with the dialysis patients attending to their needs. Theirs is a demanding job which means life or death for people who have no other alternative to dialysis. Since a dialysis clinic is off limits to the public, due to the risk of infection to patients, few people are aware of the role these professionals play in the lives of so many.

My regular doctor had now turned my care over to my nephrologist (a kidney specialist) who would be my primary doctor moving forward. I asked him questions each time I had the opportunity in order to learn as much as possible about dialysis and ways I could make life at home better for the two of us. I continued dialysis at the hemo-dialysis clinic. This method of dialysis is given this name since blood (hemoglobin, hemo) is filtered by a dialysis machine. My doctor mentioned one day that he thought I would be an excellent candidate for "peritoneal dialysis." Of course, I had to ask what that meant since I had no idea. He explained that we each have what is referred to as a "third kidney." This so-called third kidney is actually our peritoneum, a membrane within our stomach cavity which can act as a filter to remove waste from our body. This form of dialysis is referred to as peritoneal dialysis. He said he would schedule an appointment with a specially trained nurse who would explain the peritoneal dialysis process and also be my instructor. I was eager to try anything which would free me from the clinic environment, so a meeting with the nurse was scheduled. She began our first session by showing illustrations of the process and also a short film of a man undergoing peritoneal dialysis. It was something new to me since I had never heard the term, "peritoneal dialysis." She was very thorough as she explained how the body pulls fluid through the peritoneum and leaves impurities behind in the dialysis fluid to be discarded.

    She explained that a tube would be surgically implanted into my lower abdomen before I could discontinue hemo-dialysis at the clinic. One end of the tube would extend through the skin to allow dialysis fluid to fill my stomach cavity at regular intervals, four times each day, and remain until the next "exchange." The solution is pulled through the peritoneum during the "dwell" time, cleaning the blood during the process. This is, of course, a very simplistic explanation of a somewhat complex process. The true name for this process is manual peritoneal dialysis. It is called this since the patient actually performs the exchanges. After thinking and reading about peritoneal dialysis for a few days, I decided this system might be a much better alternative than having to visit the dialysis center and sit for the required four hours, three times each week. Peritoneal dialysis would be four times each day, seven days per week, but I could do this at home and have at least some freedom between "exchanges."After surgery to have the tube placed in my lower abdomen and a short recovery time, I was ready to begin peritoneal dialysis training. I would then begin dialysis at home. The access port remained in my chest in case I needed to return to the clinic for hemo-dialysis. I did not stay on hemo-dialysis long enough to require a "fistula," which is another surgery joining an artery to a vein, usually in the arm, for hemo-dialysis.

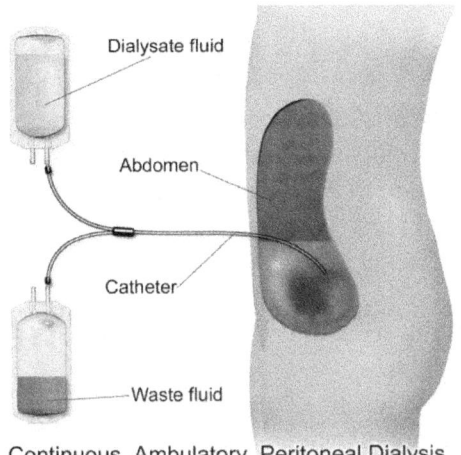

Very basic illustration of peritoneal dialysis
Courtesy Wiki-commons

I had been taught that I could expect one exchange process to take approximately forty minutes from start to finish. I soon discovered that I could not get my exchange process completed in less than ninety minutes no matter how I tried. The fluid was slow to fill and also slow to drain. It was suggested that I stand, but that didn't make it work any faster. I would try lying down with the bag of fluid hanging high overhead, but it still took much too long. I was extremely frustrated by the time I finished an exchange since it was then nearly time to begin another. I was spending all my waking hours completing fluid exchanges. I began to wonder if I had made the right decision about changing to this type of dialysis.

I felt as if I was tied to the pole holding the fluid bag. After a lot of discussion, it was decided that the tube placed in my abdomen had been placed in a poor position, causing it to drain much too slowly. I could not have a second operation to have the tube relocated due to the additional scar tissue. I would have to make the best I could with this situation or go back to the dialysis center. I decided I would rather deal with this latest problem rather than return to the dialysis center. After some time had passed the process did seem to take less time, perhaps due to a change in the positioning of the tube.

Continuing with peritoneal dialysis at home also meant changes to our home as well. Peritoneal home dialysis requires boxes of dialysis solution and accompanying tubes, bags, and other supplies to be delivered each month. Each delivery contained the supplies for the following month and required a heated and cooled location for storage. We dedicated one room inside our home to storage. Cases of fluid and supplies were stacked high each month taking up space. The large number of empty cardboard boxes also created a disposal problem as well.

Since we had stepping stones from our front entrance, a new sidewalk had to be poured so the driver could use his powered hand trucks to get the supplies into our house. I learned to do the four daily fluid exchanges as a part of my new life. Some people thought that I only had to do this procedure once each day and were surprised to learn it had to be done four times daily, seven days each week. I certainly didn't enjoy peritoneal dialysis, but I didn't have but one other alternative. I was determined to make the best of my new situation.

After I had grown somewhat accustomed to this new lifestyle, I began to wonder just how much actual living I could do while on peritoneal dialysis. At my next doctor visit, I asked for his thoughts about me taking a ship cruise. We had gone on a cruise before dialysis and really enjoyed the experience. I was ready for a change of scenery, and I thought perhaps going on a cruise while on dialysis would be a positive challenge. I needed to prove I could find some enjoyment in life and continue with this daily routine. I needed to do this for my mental health as well.

After thinking a moment, he gave his approval if I could work out the arrangements with the cruise line. I phoned the cruise line when I came home and explained my situation, and the representative assured me they would work with me and help in any way possible. At that point I was ready to go.

Our cruise ship was to leave from Jacksonville, Florida. A special courier from Orlando was to deliver the boxes of dialysis supplies to the ship terminal. I had been assured by the dialysis supply company that those supplies would be there before the ship sailed. I was solely responsible for my dialysis supplies traveling to and from the ship. One problem I had to overcome was finding a way to warm the solution since I could not take any type of warming appliance on board due to fire and safety regulations. We purchased a twelve-volt appliance which heated and cooled so that I could use it in the car or motel room, but I could not take it on the ship. Knowing the shower water on the ship was very hot, I purchased a folding cooler to use as a water container. Before doing an exchange, I filled the container with hot water and placed the bag of solution inside about thirty minutes before needed.

When we arrived at the cruise terminal in Jacksonville, we went to the check-in desk, and I gave the attendant our names. The lady looked up at me with eyes open wide, realizing I was the passenger who had been flagged on her computer screen. She was well aware of my situation and knew about the necessity of getting the supplies on board before sailing.

She asked us to please take a seat in a special area designated as "VIP," and I didn't know why, but I liked being in the VIP area. I had never gotten to sit in a VIP section before that day. She explained that I would not be allowed to board the ship until the dialysis supplies were actually placed in our room. I assured her that I did not want to leave port until I knew those supplies were on board, and we continued to wait patiently for further word.

In a while she came to let us know the courier had arrived and the dialysis supplies were being transported to the ship. It would not be long until we would be boarding. I had begun to worry the supplies might not arrive in time, but her news helped relieve my stress.

I felt better knowing things were going as planned. A gentleman in a cruise line sport coat came over to us and said our area would be first to board. I had never been a VIP before and (I have never been one since), but I did like the feeling as we walked up the ramp ahead of the other eighteen hundred people behind us, waiting their turn to be called. Had I been given the choice, I would rather have not been in the VIP section and not been on dialysis. I learned later that people actually pay for the privilege of sitting in that area to avoid the large line of people boarding. We were VIPS and didn't even have to pay! We first went to our room and then to the lido deck where we had something to drink and relaxed as we watched other passengers come on board. We were on a five-day cruise and enjoyed it greatly. To be out in the warm fresh air and enjoy the sea made me forget that I was dealing with dialysis and kidney failure. The people we ate with each night could not believe I was on a cruise and dialysis at the same time. I had a hard time believing it myself. I carefully chose what I ate and I made sure not to overeat. There is the misconception that one must overeat when on a cruise ship. This is not true. Some of the best meals I have ever eaten are those served in the ship restaurants, elegantly prepared with smaller portions and elegantly served. I did not eat at the buffet bars, the all-night pizza bars, and endless food offerings. It is up to the individual to make good decisions concerning food.

We had a great time on that cruise and have also gone on others since then. I learned that I could adapt my dialysis routine to enjoy at least some of the things I had hoped to experience. I knew my time at the lake would now be different since I could not get in the water with a rubber tube protruding from by belly and run the risk of infection, but I could at least enjoy driving our boat and seeing the lake. Life was changing, and I was trying hard to adapt.

I had begun dialysis in July of 2008 and it was then into late fall. I was using the peritoneal dialysis "manual" method, which meant I had to do the four daily exchanges following a schedule each day. I learned that a variation of this procedure was possible using a machine called a "cycler." This machine would actually perform these fluid exchanges as I slept. The official name for this dialysis method is "automated peritoneal dialysis". I began to read about this method, and it seemed a better alternative since the dialysis could be done during the night and allow me more freedom during the day. The diet restrictions would still remain the same along with the tube in my abdomen, but it seemed a better alternative to me.

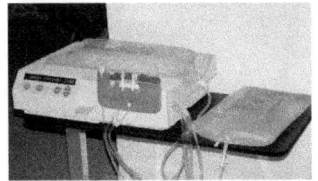

Automatic peritoneal dialysis machine. . . . my "cycler"

I had to receive additional training to learn how to use the machine. This is a miraculous invention which is a very high tech piece of equipment invented by the same man who gave us the Segway scooter. His inventions are intended to help those with medical problems to make their lives better. That was the original idea behind the Segway scooter, although it has been adapted for other purposes. The "cycler" has to perform several tasks in order to provide dialysis. These include warming the bag of solution mixture so it will be comfortable when it enters the abdomen. If is is too cold, it causes pain and discomfort. The machine must also drain and fill the fluid at specified intervals. All this has to be done quietly to not interfere with the patient's sleep. They must be done in a closed system to prevent any form of bacteria from entering the abdominal cavity possibly causing peritonitis, a very painful condition sometimes difficult to cure. I was fortunate that I never had to deal with this additional medical condition. Since the dialysis fluid is a solution containing, of all things, a sugar -based mixture, each bag adds additional calories resulting in weight gain. Within a few months I had blossomed to about 220 pounds which put me in the obese category. I was gaining weight from the extra calories I was absorbing from the dialysis solution, I was not gaining weight from the amount of food I was eating.

Although this system has its limitations, I could still be at home and avoid the long hours sitting at the dialysis clinic. I found the nighttime cycler machine to be a marvel of engineering. No matter how advanced technology becomes, however, it can never replace our own kidneys.

Chapter 10

Moving forward . . .

My new life with dialysis began the past July and a lot of things had changed. I continued to exercise at a facility near home and do what I could, but it was minimal at best. I walked on a treadmill and used a few of the sitting machines to work my arms and legs a little, but I would tire easily. Carrying the extra weight I had gained made me lethargic. I tried to follow the dialysis-approved list of foods which I found difficult to do. Due to the severe diet restrictions, it was difficult to have any variety of foods. I always enjoyed fresh pineapple, and it is an approved dialysis food since it is low in phosphate. I have since lost my love for pineapple since I ate it so much. I had learned to associate it with dialysis. I guess it is strictly a mental image problem I developed.

My nephrologist began to encourage me about applying for a kidney transplant. At that time I was then fifty-nine years old, and I could not imagine a person my age being offered a kidney since there are so many younger people waiting for a donor to become available. I really thought he was telling me this to bolster my mental attitude. I truly didn't consider this to be realistic at all. I agreed and did the necessary paperwork with the University of Alabama in Birmingham to begin the process of becoming an organ recipient. There is much more to receiving an organ donation than simply getting on a list. The first thing I had to do was get an individual letter from my dermatologist, dentist, and urologist stating that I did not have any form of cancer. I had to provide the images from a current colonoscopy showing that I was cancer-free also. Each doctor provided documentation in a timely manner, and I was grateful that I did not have any form of cancer.

An appointment was scheduled for November with the University of Alabama in Birmingham Kidney Transplant Center. I had to undergo stress tests and other medical procedures to make sure I was healthy enough to withstand the surgery needed for a kidney transplant. My blood was evaluated in order to determine my antibodies and blood type. I knew that I had an O positive blood type but little else.

When all the required paperwork was provided and physical testing had been completed, I was scheduled for an interview with transplant physicians who would determine if I would qualify as a transplant candidate. Each doctor had various questions about my medical history, family, and lifestyle. After being interviewed by so many individual doctors, each asking similar but somewhat different questions, I began to feel as if I was applying for a new job. Perhaps in some ways I was, as I look back upon that day. I wondered why they couldn't have interviewed me as a group, but I am sure the hospital had its reasons for doing it that way. I would suspect each doctor wanted to form an independent opinion of each patient's potential as an organ recipient.

Due to my ignorance of organ transplantation protocol, I asked one of the doctors, "If I qualify for a kidney, how long can I expect to be on a waiting list?"

"Three to five years," he replied. I did not get my hopes up, knowing that was a long time. I was fifty-nine years old after all, and I knew there were probably a lot of younger people on the waiting list already. My wife and I had gone through a lot of testing and evaluations to get to this point; I felt it had probably been of little use. We came back home, and I continued my same routine, nightly dialysis hooked to a peritoneal dialysis machine. I still had two problems to deal with, one was the diabetes which meant monitoring blood glucose and trying to keep blood sugar under some kind of control. The other problem, of course, was the kidney failure and dialysis. It almost seemed the two problems worked against each other as I tried to manage a balancing act between the two. I could eat some items which made the dialysis easier, but some of those items caused my blood sugar to go sky-high. Pineapple is a good example since it is low in phosphate, making it healthy for dialysis, but eating pineapple very much raised my blood sugar due to the natural sugar it contains. Living in this way was a daily challenge.

At fifty-nine years old I felt I had already lived a long life. I had been able to enjoy a lot of things during my life that so many people would never have had the opportunity to do. I had been able to work with kids during my career in public education, and I never thought of anything I would rather have done. I had been fortunate to work in a good school system which had wonderful local support from a community that valued public education. I was so fortunate to have had such support in so many ways. I had a great family, a super-supportive wife and a grown, successful son. We had enjoyed our weekends at the lake many years with friends and family, I felt I had been a very fortunate man. I knew so many people who had never achieved fifty-nine years of life. I had known kids who had died of various causes much too early, and I had seen so many other people who had dealt with personal challenges much greater than mine which limited their personal freedom and lifestyle. I resigned to make the best of my situation, but I felt I would not have the three to five years needed for a transplant.

I completed the interview process in November and was soon notified that I had been approved to be added to the kidney transplant waiting list. Many people do not realize that we can live quite well with only one kidney. There are those who were actually born with only one kidney and didn't discover that until later in life. Studies have shown that people who donate a kidney do not shorten their life by even one day. In my case, I had no family member available as a donor. My wife offered, but due to her age, she was not considered a good candidate. My only option was to wait until an anonymous donor organ became available.

I continued my home dialysis routine each night, and it had then become April of the next year following my transplant interview in November. I had prepared the machine for the night and had been on dialysis about thirty minutes in order to get in the required hours of dialysis before morning. When the phone rang at 8:30, my wife answered to discover that my sister-in-law was frantic. She had been contacted by the transplant unit in Birmingham saying they needed to get in touch with me. Alice had been on the phone for a long while, and they had contacted my sister-in-law since she was our back up emergency phone contact. I immediately called the Birmingham unit but had no idea why they would be calling me at that time of night. I thought perhaps they had found something new about my blood work, or I needed to update some information. I had been told I could expect to wait three to five years for a transplant, and it had been less than six months since being told that, so I could not imagine anything further.

When the young man answered in Birmingham I told him who I was and asked why he had called. He said, "We want you here by midnight."

Still clueless, I asked, "Why?"

He said, "You are getting a kidney . . . and a pancreas." I sat back, caught my breath for a moment and tried to think of questions to ask, but I was so surprised I really could not think of any. I finally thanked him for calling and assured him I would be there. What a night this would turn out to be. Once again my life was going to undergo another major change. I knew this was not a sure thing, but I had to think positively.

Chapter 11

The transplant experience . . .

We each have special days during our lives that we will always remember. I will always remember where I was and what I was doing the day President John F. Kennedy was shot and killed in Dallas, Texas. I will always remember the morning I was enjoying my early morning coffee while watching the "Today Show" when the image of a burning New York skyscraper, the World Trade Center tower, appeared on the screen. Suddenly, a passenger jet appeared from the right side of the screen and crashed into the second World Trade Center tower, leaving me in a state of disbelief. I will also remember the night I received the phone call from the University of Alabama in Birmingham hospital letting me know I was in line to receive a double organ transplant. Me? Why me? I was fifty-nine years old, there surely had to be someone needier than I. It was so hard to believe. I quickly got off the phone and made a couple of calls to let some friends know what I had just learned and that we would be leaving for Birmingham very soon. We hurriedly tossed a few clothes and toiletries together, locked the door behind us and headed south toward Birmingham. We had less than three hours to get to Birmingham, plenty of time in most cases, but I could imagine a back up on the interstate, or perhaps a flat tire or other mechanical failure which would cause us to arrive there past our deadline. I had to ask my wife to slow down as she drove along the interstate, fearing she was likely to see blue lights pulling us over for a speeding ticket. I could understand her stress; I felt stressed, too, but I tried to keep mine under control and not add to hers. We had lots to discuss as we cruised down the interstate, not knowing anything more than what I learned during the earlier phone call. What would I experience during the operation? How long would it take to recover? The reality of the situation finally began to sink in.

We arrived in Birmingham and hurriedly ran to the emergency room to check in as instructed on the phone. As soon as I had signed in and provided insurance information, I was whisked away from the emergency room to a standard hospital room to begin preparing for surgery. I did not realize it at that time, but they did not want me to linger in the emergency room waiting area for fear that I might contract some sort of virus or infection which might put my surgery in jeopardy.

The first staff member I met was a nice lady named Pat who gave me a thin hospital gown and asked me to put it on. I did so and came back to lie on the bed as she told me what was to happen next. Three hours earlier I had been at home preparing for bed, attached to my dialysis machine. I was now in a hospital gown in downtown Birmingham in the middle of the night, unaware of the events to come. Pat explained that I would need to have my stomach and intestines emptied before surgery. This may be standard surgery protocol and I won't go into great detail, but let me say it involved a long tube and lots and lots of water . . . repeatedly. Pat and I came to know each other quite well. When this procedure was completed, an IV was inserted, blood was drawn and other personnel came in to check on me and perform their duties. I began to feel much like a pin cushion due to all the needles and finger pricks as they monitored my blood sugar and kidney function. Since I had to quickly stop my dialysis earlier that night, my creatnine level was extremely high. Creatnine is the waste product the kidneys filter from the blood. A normal creatnine reading is between .7 and 1.3. My creatnine level that night was 13, about thirteen times higher than a normal reading. As the night wore on, I kept wondering how much longer I would be waiting before surgery began. I did not realize at that time that medical personnel were probably doing everything in their power to save someone's life in another part of the hospital. When all efforts fail and an organ donor dies, another group of doctors trained in organ recovery work just as hard to preserve precious organs in order to help someone in need. I had no idea how the system worked, and I was only thinking about myself. By daybreak I was still waiting and growing hungry and thirsty since I had not been given anything to eat and very little water during the entire night. It seemed I needed to be ready for surgery at any time, and they could not take the chance of giving me anything to eat or drink.

    The morning passed, and I continued to wait for further instructions. At about two o'clock in the afternoon someone came into the room and announced that they were ready to take me to surgery. By this time I had grown weak from not eating and really felt quite relieved having waited all night and most of the next day to begin surgery. My primary surgeon had visited with me earlier to discuss the risks associated with this major surgery and wanted me to realize that it came with associated risks, one of which was death. I assured him I was aware of the risk, and I was willing to accept that risk, knowing that I was not happy with being tied to a machine each night for dialysis and the associated problems that came along with it. I was resigned to accept whatever happened.

    I was wheeled into a room near the operating room and final preparations were made. I said goodbye to my wife, said, "I love you," and that was the last thing I remember about that day. I was confident that I was in the care of some very skilled and caring surgeons and staff. Within a short time, three well trained and talented surgeons began the task of giving me a new kidney and pancreas.

    When I awoke nine hours later, I immediately began to look at my surroundings, trying to make sense of them. I won't go into further details about my post surgery experiences, but the first day in recovery was rough since I could not move. I was still not allowed to have anything to eat or drink for fear that I would become sick and throw up, possibly tearing my long incision or ripping something inside my abdomen. Each day after became a little easier as I became accustomed to the hospital routine. I tried to make myself a little stronger by walking as much as I could. Those walks were very measured as I dragged my IV pole along beside me.

The new kidney was placed in my abdomen on the left side. The pancreas was placed in my abdomen on the right side. Both were working perfectly. An illustration shows the location of the new pancreas and kidney. My own kidneys and pancreas were left in place so I now have three kidneys and two pancreases. Until the night of my transplant surgery, I was on dialysis in order to stay alive. The following day after surgery I did not require dialysis and the large volume of fluid I was holding began to be drawn from my body. My weight began to drop toward my normal range in a very few days. I had soon lost forty pounds. The pancreas was producing insulin and the insulin shots I had been giving myself for thirty-five years were no longer needed. I felt as if I was beginning my life again. I almost felt as if I had become twenty-four once more.

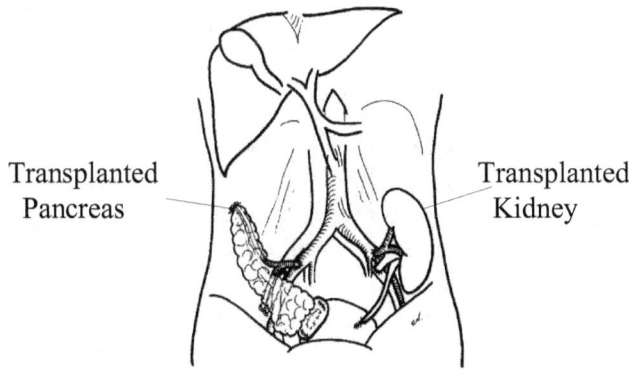

Transplanted Pancreas

Transplanted Kidney

After two very long weeks in the hospital, I was moved to a nearby hospital town house so anti rejection medications could be monitored daily. I had to return to the lab each morning at six-thirty to have blood drawn, but I could then return to the townhouse for the rest of the day. Life was beginning to return to some form of normalcy after a few weeks. I was soon permitted to come home for weekends which allowed me to sleep in my bed once again. Within several weeks I was released to come home completely. I was still required to return to Birmingham quite often in order to have medication levels checked as well as my overall condition.

There is not one day which passes that I do not think how fortunate I am to have been an organ recipient. I realize that I possibly would not be here today had I not received the transplant. Thirty-five years with diabetes was suddenly gone. The injections and needle prick, gone. The need to constantly monitor my diet in order to maintain blood sugar control was also gone. The dialysis and extreme diet restrictions, gone as well. I definitely continue to monitor my diet and work to maintain a proper weight but not to the extreme that was required to for so many years. I occasionally eat a piece of pie without the feeling of guilt that I once had. I no longer have to worry about the low blood sugar episodes which could send me to the hospital emergency room. Most people consider getting older to be a curse, in my case I felt as if I was actually getting younger instead. I felt that way both mentally and physically.

It has now been more than five years since receiving my transplants, and these have probably been the best five years of my life. I don't think I knew how to appreciate my good health so many years earlier. I try to visit the gym and exercise each day, I still do not smoke and I feel great. I have received great lab reports during these five years, and I have not encountered any indication of rejection. Should these organs fail, I want it to be due to something beyond my control. I try to follow my doctor's orders as closely as I possibly can. I know I will never be given this very special gift ever again. There are so many people who need a kidney, liver, or other organ who will never live long enough to obtain one. Perhaps one day we will have the ability to provide needed organs in some manner other than organ donation, but until that day arrives I encourage everyone to become an organ donor, especially younger people. It makes no sense to put healthy organs into the ground when someone dies. Those same organs might help someone live a better life, or in fact, live.

1.
In 1889, Oskar Minkowski (1858-1931) discovered the link between the pancreas and insulin when a dog from which he removed the pancreas developed diabetes.

Some basic facts concerning organ donation from the United Network for Organ Sharing are worth noting:

1. People of all ages and medical histories should consider themselves potential donors. Your medical condition at the time of death will determine what organs and tissue can be donated.

2. Organs and tissues that can be donated include: heart, kidneys, lungs, pancreas, liver, intestines, corneas, skin, tendons, bone, and heart valve.

3. There is no national registry of organ donors. Even if you have indicated your wishes on your driver's license or a donor card, be sure you have told your family as they will be consulted before donation can take place.

4. All major religions approve of organ and tissue donation and consider donation the greatest gift.

5. An open casket funeral is possible for organ and tissue donors.

There are firm rules which must be followed about contact between the organ donor's family and the organ recipient. Both the donor's family and the recipient must agree to have contact with the other party, and contact is monitored through an organization called the United Network for Organ Sharing. One year must pass before any correspondence between parties can be exchanged and then only through this organization. I gave my written permission to be contacted, and the mother of the deceased young man had also. A little more than one year had passed when one day I received my copy of a special letter which had been written to provide the same information to those who had received organs from this lady's son,

Bobby. I had been given a kidney and pancreas, I could only imagine that someone else had received the other kidney and other lifesaving organs. I could only imagine. I had no knowledge other than my own involvement.

As I opened the envelope, I noticed an attached page written in block letters as one might expect from a younger elementary student. This page of the letter was from his seven-year-old daughter. She wrote from her heart about her father and ended by saying she had blue eyes just like her daddy. I would be lying if I said reading this did not affect me emotionally. I could not speak as I read the letter, I found it extremely difficult to control my emotions when finally my wife began to ask me questions and I could only hand the letter to her to read. The other letter was from Bobby's mother which provided information about her son. She wrote that he had a love for motorcycle riding and a kind heart, always wanting to help others. Being an organ donor was just one additional way he could do that. I could only imagine the grief this mother must have felt as she wrote this letter. I could not help but feel guilt when I thought that at that time I was fifty-nine years old, and Bobby had died at the age of thirty-three with so much of his life before him. I had enjoyed a great life already. I think of his little girl often and try to imagine how she might have grown and matured since I received her letter.

> When matching donor organs to recipients, the computerized matching system considers issues such as the severity of the illness, blood type, time spent waiting, other important medical information, and geographical location. The recipient's financial or celebrity status or race does not figure in.

Chapter 12

A new lease on life . . .

As I lay in my hospital bed during recovery, I began to realize just how fortunate I had been to receive this new lease on life, particularly at my age. I had lots of time to think, and I began to formulate a plan to become as healthy as I possibly could when I was able to go home. I could now enjoy a new life free from insulin injections thanks to the new pancreas, and without dialysis thanks to the new kidney.

My doctors encouraged me to maintain a healthy weight since doing so would help the new organs function better and hopefully last many years longer. I would be required to take anti rejection drugs for the remainder of my life, but swallowing a few pills each day seemed a small price to pay after thirty-five years of daily multiple insulin injections and the rigors of kidney dialysis. The medical staff kept letting me know how important it was to always take the anti rejection medication, I assured them that I would certainly do so. I would follow their orders. I knew how important the medication was to my overall health. I could not understand how some organ recipients ignore their anti rejection medicine and lose their transplanted organs.

I made the decision to improve my diet and eat as healthily as possible. I wanted to eat more green vegetables and natural fruits and avoid the "junk" food which I feel is causing problems for so many people today, especially the very young. I do not drink soft drinks at all anymore. When I was diabetic, I drank diet soft drinks, not too many, but I did drink them.

With dialysis, diet drinks are not allowed due to the phosphate and salt which they contain. Since phosphate is hard to remove with dialysis, I decided it might not be good for the new kidney as well. Regular soft drinks are laden with sugar, so they only help to add extra pounds and provide no food value. I have not had a soft drink in five years, and I don't miss them. I drink tea, coffee, or water instead. I try to control my weight by watching portions and making good dietary choices.

    I go online before eating out to check the online menu and know before I reach the restaurant exactly what I will order. I can quickly give my order to the waitress and watch as others study the menu to make menu decisions. The waiters and waitresses seem to like my approach, since it saves them time. I have learned to enjoy salads with a protein topping, the kind of salad which is made with the healthy Romaine lettuce and a variety of vegetables. I search for the grilled items (the grilled shrimp, chicken, or grilled vegetables) rather than those fried. I avoid fried foods due to the extra fat and calories.

    I continue to exercise each day at an exercise facility. I learned long ago that exercising alone did not work well for me. I enjoy being in the company of those who also want to be healthier. When I dress to exercise, I feel I have put on my "uniform" and have made some sort of commitment to take part. I do not exercise in a group, but just being with others exercising helps to improve my spirit and mood. I do not belong to a "gym" with muscle-bound men lifting weights trying to prove their youthfulness, but instead I work out at a facility where many people have experienced physical problems and are working to make themselves as healthy as possible once again. When I look around while there, I see people who have had major surgeries, knee replacements, or other health problems. It helps me to realize I am not the only person who has had problems. My daily routine usually consists of stretching and twenty or thirty minutes on an elliptical machine during which time I burn between

250 and 400 calories depending upon the amount of time I am on the machine. I do more weight training on Monday, Wednesday and Friday with less time on the elliptical machine. The last thing I do each day is finish by doing twenty-five pushups. This routine seems to work for me, and I don't have to spend my entire day at the facility. So far my lab reports during these five years have been excellent, I believe my approach to diet and exercise has worked well for me. My ideal Body Mass Index score would be a weight of 159. I seem to stay just over that goal with a weight of 165 or 166 during summer and about 168 during winter. Too much time indoors with too much comfort food is hard for me to resist. In warmer weather I can find a variety of outdoor activities to burn off the extra calories. I try to do the best I can, but I am far from perfect.

While enjoying my early morning coffee on another recent cruise, I had the opportunity to talk with a fellow passenger who shared a story with me about his step son, a twenty-four-year-old young man who had been living with juvenile, type one, diabetes since the age of five. He told how the step son had become defensive about having to maintain his rigorous lifestyle with the constant blood sugar monitoring and attention to diet and all the additional worries that come with this condition. I could understand the young man's feelings probably more that most, but even I could not imagine the life this young man had lived before reaching the age of twenty-four. I had been around twenty-four when I was diagnosed with diabetes, he had been dealing with diabetes for nearly twenty years before he reached the age of twenty-four. His step father said the young man was tired of his mother reminding him to self-monitor his blood sugar and also reminding him about what to eat, or not to eat. I could understand that also. At that time of his life he should have been experiencing a carefree lifestyle, eating with friends, and partying. Instead, he had to worry about blood sugar, and making excuses why he could not eat the foods his friends could enjoy. He also had to deal with the feeling that he did not fit in. At some time, I had experienced those same feelings. It isn't fair, and I am sure he felt that life had not treated him fairly as well. If I could have talked with the young man, I would have suggested that he read about diabetes and work to keep himself as healthy as possible. No one knows when scientific advances are coming to make type one diabetes disappear. Advances in stem cell research are currently making headlines, and perhaps it will soon be possible to transplant the cells which make insulin. It can happen, but these advances don't usually happen overnight. Research takes time and money. If he is as healthy as possible, he may be a good candidate for a pancreas transplant or some device which will make life with diabetes easier. It is so hard to realize that what we do today is so important to our future when it comes to preventing diabetic complications.

Those who have type two diabetes are not immune from the same complications that are caused by type one diabetes. A poorly controlled glucose level with type two diabetes is just as damaging as with type one. Those individuals should take their medical condition seriously and try to maintain good blood sugar levels also.

Since type two diabetes can often be prevented, I felt I should include some information that people might find useful. I also included information about gestational diabetes since that form of diabetes is often overlooked.

I found the National Diabetes Education Program to be an excellent source of free information for those with either type one or type two diabetes. The following booklet is a great resource for those hoping to decrease their chances of having type two diabetes in the future.

"Your Game Plan to Prevent Type Two Diabetes"

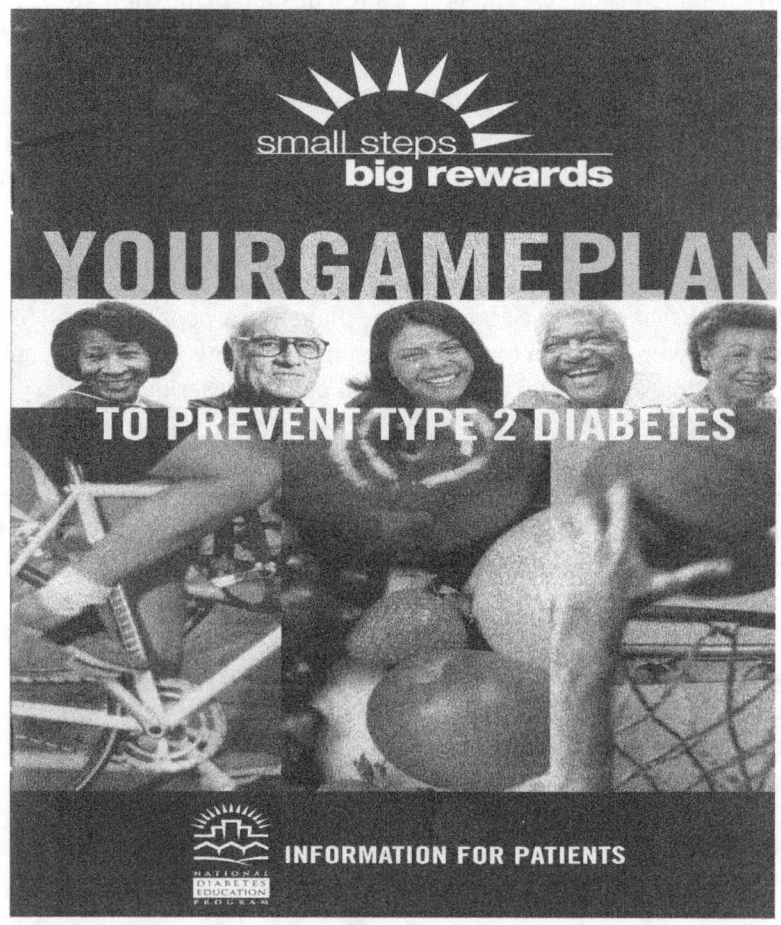

Are you at risk for diabetes?

Are You At-Risk Check List

Find out if you are at risk for diabetes and pre-diabetes.
There are many factors that increase your risk for diabetes. To find out about your risk, check each item that applies to you.

- ☐ I am 45 years of age or older.

- ☐ The At-Risk Weight Chart on page 15 that shows my current weight puts me at risk.

- ☐ I have a parent, brother, or sister with diabetes.

- ☐ My family background is African American, Hispanic/Latino, American Indian, Asian American, or Pacific Islander.

- ☐ I have had diabetes while I was pregnant (this is called gestational diabetes) or I gave birth to a baby weighing 9 pounds or more.

- ☐ I have been told that my glucose levels are higher than normal.

- ☐ My blood pressure is 140/90 or higher, or I have been told that I have high blood pressure.

- ☐ My cholesterol (lipid) levels are not normal. My HDL cholesterol ("good" cholesterol) is less than 35 or my triglyceride level is higher than 250.

Almost 21 million Americans have diabetes—one-third don't even know it. You need to know if you are at risk for diabetes.

continued on next pages. . . .

-87-

....continued from a previous page . . .

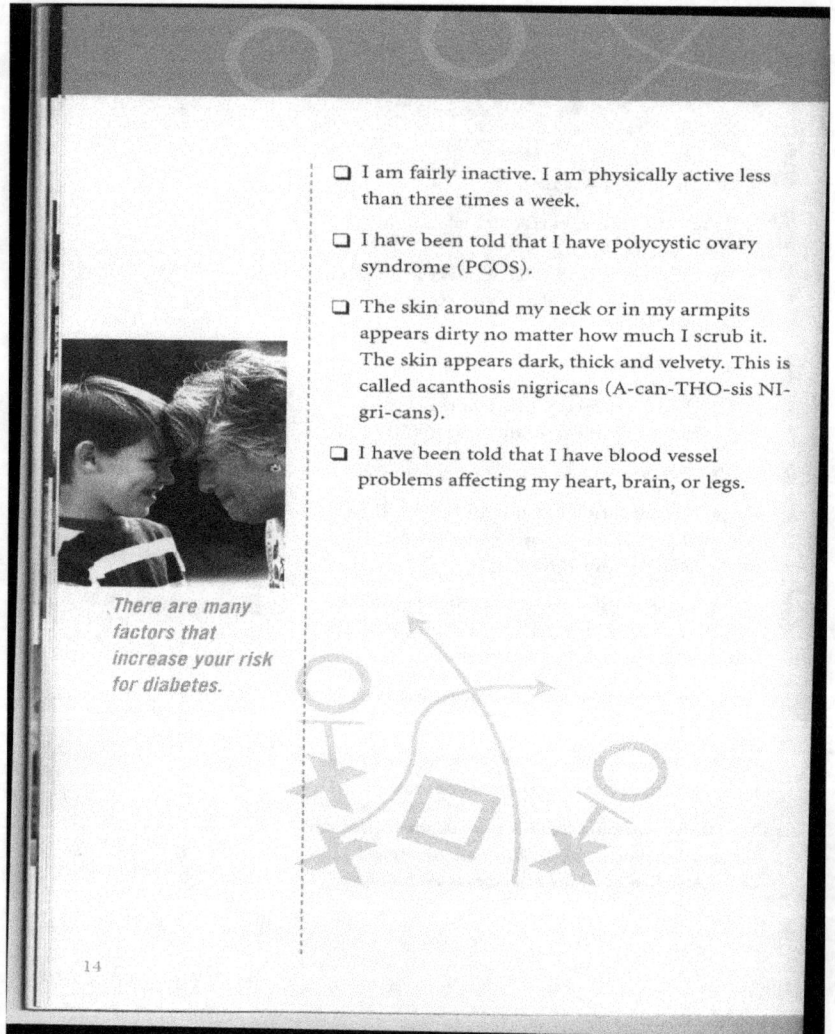

- ❏ I am fairly inactive. I am physically active less than three times a week.
- ❏ I have been told that I have polycystic ovary syndrome (PCOS).
- ❏ The skin around my neck or in my armpits appears dirty no matter how much I scrub it. The skin appears dark, thick and velvety. This is called acanthosis nigricans (A-can-THO-sis NI-gri-cans).
- ❏ I have been told that I have blood vessel problems affecting my heart, brain, or legs.

There are many factors that increase your risk for diabetes.

The following page provides further information about the questionnaire.

If you have checked any of the items, a follow-up health check is recommended . . .

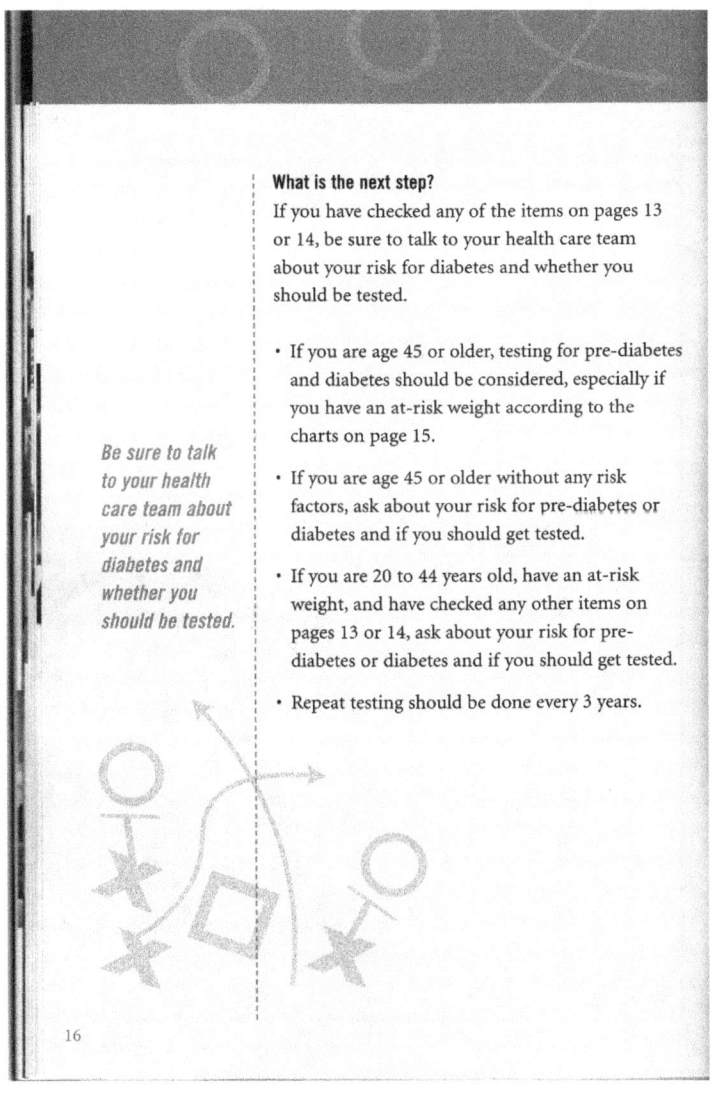

What is the next step?

If you have checked any of the items on pages 13 or 14, be sure to talk to your health care team about your risk for diabetes and whether you should be tested.

- If you are age 45 or older, testing for pre-diabetes and diabetes should be considered, especially if you have an at-risk weight according to the charts on page 15.

- If you are age 45 or older without any risk factors, ask about your risk for pre-diabetes or diabetes and if you should get tested.

- If you are 20 to 44 years old, have an at-risk weight, and have checked any other items on pages 13 or 14, ask about your risk for pre-diabetes or diabetes and if you should get tested.

- Repeat testing should be done every 3 years.

Be sure to talk to your health care team about your risk for diabetes and whether you should be tested.

The following free materials are from the National Diabetes Education Program.

...for those concerned with gestational diabetes . . .

ENGLISH

Did You Have Gestational Diabetes When You Were Pregnant?

What You Need to Know.

Some women get diabetes when they are pregnant. Doctors call this gestational (jes-TAY-shun-al) diabetes. Most of the time, it goes away after your baby is born. Even if the diabetes goes away, you still have a greater chance of getting diabetes later in life. Your child may also have a greater chance of being obese and getting type 2 diabetes later in life. Use this tip sheet to learn what you can do for yourself and your child.

Action steps for you

Get tested for diabetes:

- Get tested for diabetes 6 to 12 weeks after your baby is born. If the test is normal, get tested every 3 years. If the test results show that your blood sugar (glucose) is higher than normal but not high enough to be diabetes, also called prediabetes, get tested for diabetes every year.
- Talk to your doctor about your test results and what you can do to stay healthy.
- If your test results show that you could get diabetes and you are overweight, ask your doctor about what changes you can make to lose weight and for help in making them. You may need to take medicine such as metformin to help prevent type 2 diabetes.

NDEP — National Diabetes Education Program
A program of the National Institutes of Health and the Centers for Disease Control and Prevention

...further information about gestational diabetes.

Change the foods you eat and be more active:

- Choose healthy foods such as:
  - fruits that are fresh, frozen, or canned in water
  - lean meats, chicken and turkey with the skin removed, and fish
  - skim or low-fat milk, cheese, and yogurt
  - vegetables, whole grains, dried beans, and peas
- Drink water instead of juice and regular soda.
- Eat smaller amounts of food to help you reach and stay at a healthy weight. For example, eat a 3-ounce hamburger instead of a 6-ounce hamburger. Three ounces is about the size of your fist or a deck of cards.
- Be more active each day. Try to get at least 30 minutes of activity, 5 days a week. It is okay to be active for 10 minutes at a time, 3 times a day. Walk with friends, swim, or garden to move more.
- Try to get back to a healthy weight. Talk to your health care team about a plan to help you lose weight slowly. Being at a healthy weight can help reduce your chances of getting type 2 diabetes.

Action steps for the whole family

- Ask your doctor for an eating plan that will help your children grow and be at a healthy weight.
- Help your children make healthy food choices.
- Help your children be active for at least 60 minutes each day.
- Do things together as a family, such as making healthy meals or playing active games together.
- Limit TV, video, and computer game time to an hour or two a day.
- Contact your local parks department or local health department to learn where you can find safe places to be active and get healthy foods.

Other action steps

- Tell your doctor or health care team if:
  - you had gestational diabetes
  - you want to get pregnant again
- Breastfeed your baby to help you lose weight and improve your child's health.
- Make sure your history of gestational diabetes is in your child's health record.

Things to remember:

- Get tested for diabetes 6 to 12 weeks after your baby is born.
- Take steps to lower your chances of getting diabetes by being more active and making healthy food choices.
- Help your children be healthy and lower their chances of getting type 2 diabetes.

National Diabetes Education Program
1-888-693-NDEP (1-888-693-6337) • www.YourDiabetesInfo.org

Francine R. Kaufman, M.D., Professor Emeritus of Pediatrics and Communications at the University of Southern California and attending physician at Children's Hospital Los Angeles reviewed this material for accuracy.

HHS' NDEP is jointly sponsored by NIH and CDC with the support of more than 200 partner organizations.

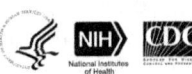

NIH Publication No. 13-6019 | NDEP-88
Revised April 2013
The NIDDK prints on recycled paper with bio-based ink.

I believe one of the most important things someone with diabetes should do is work with a doctor who is up to date on the latest developments in diabetes treatment. This field of medicine is always changing with better drugs, insulin, and technical advancements which can make a positive difference in the life of someone with diabetes. When glucose monitors became available and did not require blood from the finger tip but instead from the fleshy area of the forearm, I checked my blood sugar much more frequently. That area of the forearm has less pain sensors than the finger tip, and I didn't mind checking more often. A doctor who is not willing to listen and thinks he or she has all the answers is not necessarily the doctor I want. I searched to find a doctor with additional training in diabetes management, and I worked to form a partnership with him. Since he had someone in his immediate family with type one diabetes, I felt he would be continually trying to learn the latest information in order to help his family member. I hoped I could benefit from his interest as well.

Taking the classes offered through our local health department was one of the most beneficial things I could have done to help myself when I was first diagnosed with diabetes many years ago. Those classes were free of charge and covered so much valuable information from diet to foot care with so many areas in between. Since the classes were in a group setting, I learned that I was not the only person with concerns and questions; we were all concerned. This was uncharted territory for each of us. During those classes I came to realize how important a good diet is in the life of someone with diabetes. The "exchange diet" seems so simple now, but at first it seemed hard to understand that one food could be about the same amount of calories, fat, etc. as another and that I could "exchange" one for the other. In the class we covered the importance of checking feet to make sure there were no cuts or other problems which could lead to an infection with dangerous consequences such as amputation. I always had the image of the old gentleman in the initial doctor visit to remind me. By this age I have known too many of my friends who have developed various diabetic complications and were not as fortunate as I. Some may have tried to follow the diabetic diet and lifestyle and had problems anyway. Some, I am sure, felt immune from the long-term effects diabetes causes. I have seen the effects diabetes can have on those who disregard their health and cannot make the commitment to follow prescribed best practices. The result is not pleasant. I did not want to be one of those people.

One of the best booklets I have found is titled

4 Steps to Manage Your Diabetes for Life

This booklet contains valuable information in condensed form that anyone can easily understand. I found it worthwhile to provide a copy. Originals may be obtained from the National Diabetes Education Program free of charge. Ordering information will be provided and, it is non copyrighted material.

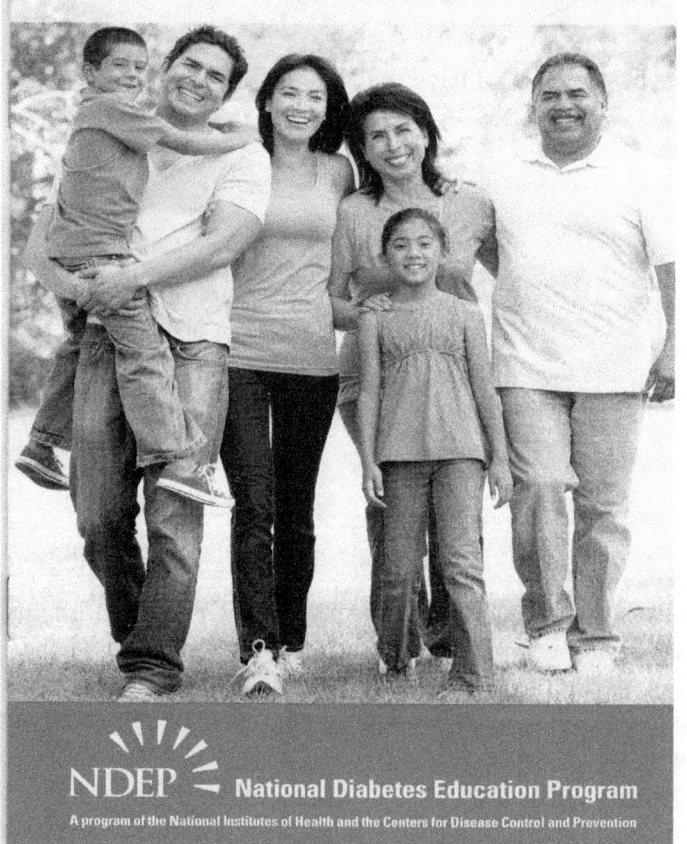

> **Actions you can take**
>
> The marks ✓ in this booklet show actions you can take to manage your diabetes.
>
> ✓ Help your health care team make a diabetes care plan that will work for you.
>
> ✓ Learn to make wise choices for your diabetes care each day.

STEP 1:
Learn about diabetes.

What is diabetes?

There are three main types of diabetes:

- Type 1 diabetes – Your body does not make insulin. This is a problem because you need insulin to take the sugar (glucose) from the foods you eat and turn it into energy for your body. You need to take insulin every day to live.
- Type 2 diabetes – Your body does not make or use insulin well. You may need to take pills or insulin to help control your diabetes. Type 2 is the most common type of diabetes.
- Gestational (jest-TAY-shun-al) diabetes – Some women get this kind of diabetes when they are pregnant. Most of the time, it goes away after the baby is born. But even if it goes away, these women and their children have a greater chance of getting diabetes later in life.

You are the most important member of your health care team.

You are the one who manages your diabetes day by day. Talk to your doctor about how you can best care for your diabetes to stay healthy. Some others who can help are:

- dentist
- diabetes doctor
- diabetes educator
- dietitian
- eye doctor
- foot doctor
- friends and family
- mental health counselor
- nurse
- nurse practitioner
- pharmacist
- social worker

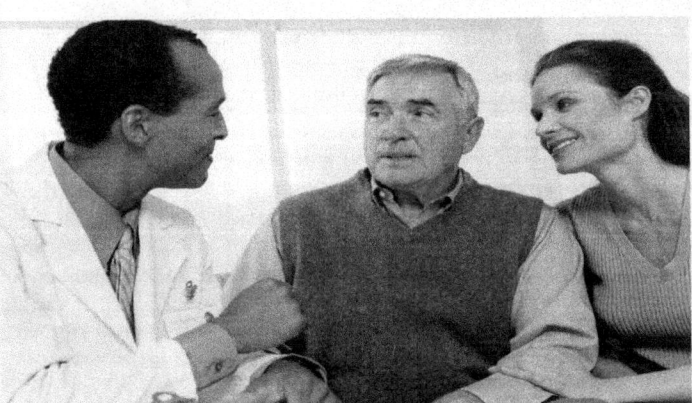

How to learn more about diabetes.

- Take classes to learn more about living with diabetes. To find a class, check with your health care team, hospital, or area health clinic. You can also search online.
- Join a support group — in-person or online — to get peer support with managing your diabetes.
- Read about diabetes online. Go to www.YourDiabetesInfo.org.

Take diabetes seriously.

You may have heard people say they have "a touch of diabetes" or that their "sugar is a little high." These words suggest that diabetes is not a serious disease. That is **not** correct. Diabetes is **serious,** but you can learn to manage it.

People with diabetes need to make healthy food choices, stay at a healthy weight, move more every day, and take their medicine even when they feel good. It's a lot to do. **It's not easy, but it's worth it!**

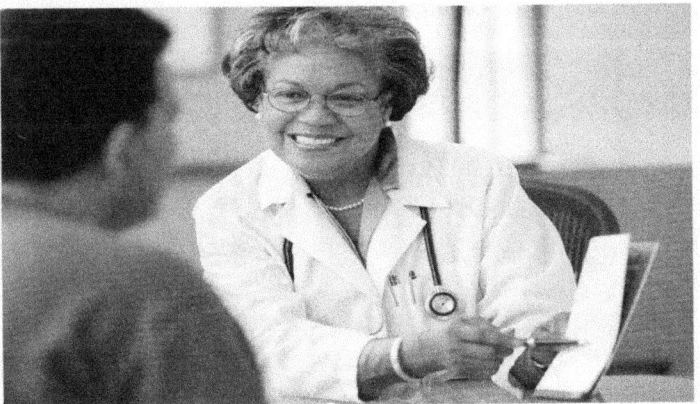

Why take care of your diabetes?

Taking care of yourself and your diabetes can help you feel good today and in the future. When your blood sugar (glucose) is close to normal, you are likely to:

- have more energy
- be less tired and thirsty
- need to pass urine less often
- heal better
- have fewer skin or bladder infections

You will also have less chance of having health problems caused by diabetes such as:

- heart attack or stroke
- eye problems that can lead to trouble seeing or going blind
- pain, tingling, or numbness in your hands and feet, also called nerve damage
- kidney problems that can cause your kidneys to stop working
- teeth and gum problems

✓ Actions you can take

- ✓ Ask your health care team what type of diabetes you have.
- ✓ Learn where you can go for support.
- ✓ Learn how caring for your diabetes helps you feel good today and in the future.

STEP 2:
Know your diabetes ABCs.

Talk to your health care team about how to manage your **A**1C, **B**lood pressure, and **C**holesterol. This can help lower your chances of having a heart attack, stroke, or other diabetes problems.

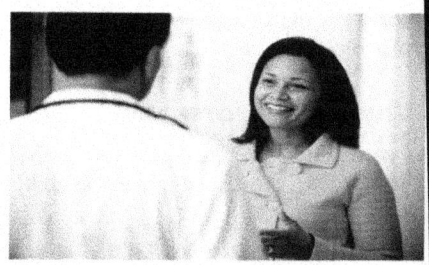

A for the A1C test (A-one-C).

What is it?

The A1C is a blood test that measures your average blood sugar level over the past three months. It is different from the blood sugar checks you do each day.

Why is it important?

You need to know your blood sugar levels over time. You don't want those numbers to get too high. High levels of blood sugar can hurt your heart and blood vessels, kidneys, feet, and eyes.

What is the A1C goal?

The A1C goal for many people with diabetes is below 7. Ask what your goal should be.

5

B for Blood pressure.

What is it?
Blood pressure is the force of your blood against the wall of your blood vessels.

Why is it important?
If your blood pressure gets too high, it makes your heart work too hard. It can cause a heart attack, stroke, and kidney disease.

What is the blood pressure goal?
The blood pressure goal for most people with diabetes is below 130/80. Ask what your goal should be.

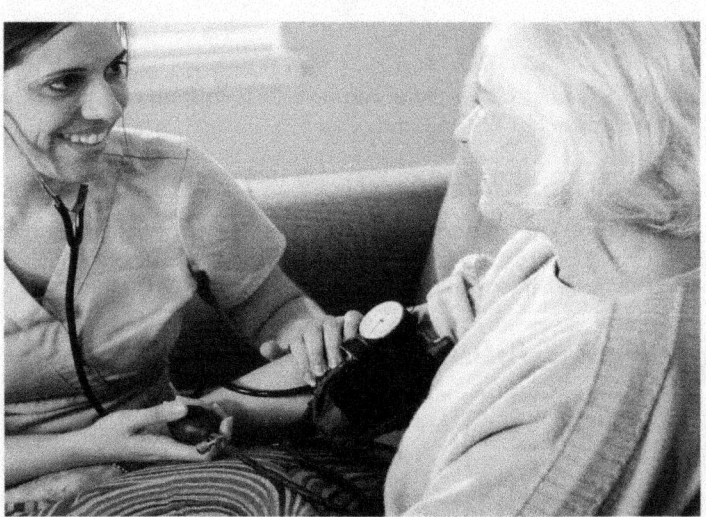

STEP 3:
Learn how to live with diabetes.

It is common to feel overwhelmed, sad, or angry when you are living with diabetes. You may know the steps you should take to stay healthy, but have trouble sticking with your plan over time. This section has tips on how to cope with your diabetes, eat well, and be active.

Cope with your diabetes.

- Stress can raise your blood sugar. Learn ways to lower your stress. Try deep breathing, gardening, taking a walk, meditating, working on your hobby, or listening to your favorite music.

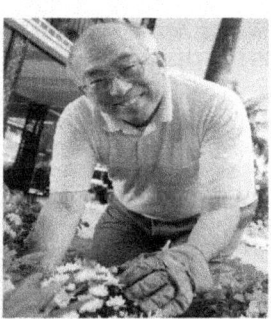

- Ask for help if you feel down. A mental health counselor, support group, member of the clergy, friend, or family member who will listen to your concerns may help you feel better.

Eat well.

- Make a diabetes meal plan with help from your health care team.
- Choose foods that are lower in calories, saturated fat, trans fat, sugar, and salt.
- Eat foods with more fiber, such as whole grain cereals, breads, crackers, rice, or pasta.
- Choose foods such as fruits, vegetables, whole grains, bread and cereals, and low-fat or skim milk and cheese.
- Drink water instead of juice and regular soda.

8

- Check your feet every day for cuts, blisters, red spots, and swelling. Call your health care team right away about any sores that do not go away.
- Brush your teeth and floss every day to keep your mouth, teeth, and gums healthy.
- Stop smoking. Ask for help to quit. Call 1-800-QUITNOW (1-800-784-8669).
- Keep track of your blood sugar. You may want to check it one or more times a day. Use the card at the back of this booklet to keep a record of your blood sugar numbers. Be sure to talk about it with your health care team.
- Check your blood pressure if your doctor advises and keep a record of it.

Talk to your health care team.
- Ask your doctor if you have any questions about your diabetes.
- Report any changes in your health.

✓ Actions you can take

✓ Ask for a healthy meal plan.

✓ Ask about ways to be more active.

✓ Ask how and when to test your blood sugar and how to use the results to manage your diabetes.

✓ Use these tips to help with your self-care.

✓ Discuss how your diabetes plan is working for you each time you visit your health care team.

STEP 4:
Get routine care to stay healthy.

See your health care team **at least twice a year** to find and treat any problems early.

At each visit, be sure you have a:

- blood pressure check
- foot check
- weight check
- review of your self-care plan

Two times each year, have an:

- A1C test. It may be checked more often if it is over 7.

Once each year, be sure you have a:

- cholesterol test
- complete foot exam
- dental exam to check teeth and gums
- dilated eye exam to check for eye problems
- flu shot
- urine and a blood test to check for kidney problems

At least once in your lifetime, get a:

- pneumonia (nu-mo-nya) shot
- hepatitis B (HEP-uh-TY-tiss) shot

Why not try to avoid having type two diabetes if possible? By making lifestyle changes, type two diabetes can actually be avoided, this is not possible with type one.

ENGLISH

Choose More than 50 Ways to Prevent Type 2 Diabetes

Learn how to prevent or delay type 2 diabetes by losing a small amount of weight. To get started, use these tips to help you move more, make healthy food choices, and track your progress.

Reduce Portion Sizes

Portion size is the amount of food you eat, such as 1 cup of fruit or 6 ounces of meat. If you are trying to eat smaller portions, eat a half of a bagel instead of a whole bagel or have a 3-ounce hamburger instead of a 6-ounce hamburger. Three ounces is about the size of your fist or a deck of cards.

Put less on your plate, Nate.

1. Drink a large glass of water 10 minutes before your meal so you feel less hungry.

2. Keep meat, chicken, turkey, and fish portions to about 3 ounces.

3. Share one dessert.

Eat a small meal, Lucille.

4. Use teaspoons, salad forks, or child-size forks, spoons, and knives to help you take smaller bites and eat less.

5. Make less food look like more by serving your meal on a salad or breakfast plate.

6. Eat slowly. It takes 20 minutes for your stomach to send a signal to your brain that you are full.

7. Listen to music while you eat instead of watching TV (people tend to eat more while watching TV).

How much should I eat?
Try filling your plate like this:

1/4 grains
1/2 vegetables and fruit
dairy (low-fat or skim milk)
1/4 protein

NDEP — National Diabetes Education Program   www.YourDiabetesInfo.org

Move More Each Day

Find ways to be more active each day. Try to be active for at least 30 minutes, 5 days a week. Walking is a great way to get started and you can do it almost anywhere at any time. Bike riding, swimming, and dancing are also good ways to move more.

If you are looking for a safe place to be active, contact your local parks department or health department to ask about walking maps, community centers, and nearby parks.

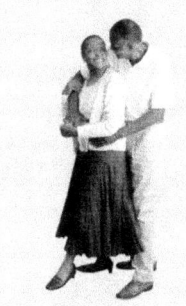

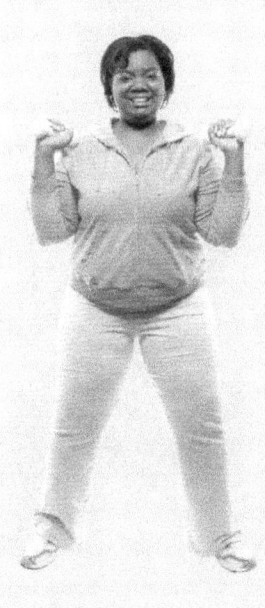

Dance it away, Faye.

8. Show your kids the dances you used to do when you were their age.

9. Turn up the music and jam while doing household chores.

10. Work out with a video that shows you how to get active.

Let's go, Flo.

11. Deliver a message in person to a co-worker instead of sending an e-mail.

12. Take the stairs to your office. Or take the stairs as far as you can, and then take the elevator the rest of the way.

13. Catch up with friends during a walk instead of by phone.

14. March in place while you watch TV.

15. Choose a place to walk that is safe, such as your local mall.

16. Get off of the bus one stop early and walk the rest of the way home or to work during the week if it is safe.

Make Healthy Food Choices

Find ways to make healthy food choices. This can help you manage your weight and lower your chances of getting type 2 diabetes.

Choose to eat more vegetables, fruits, and whole grains. Cut back on high-fat foods like whole milk, cheeses, and fried foods. This will help you reduce the amount of fat and calories you take in each day.

Snack on a veggie, Reggie.

17. Buy a mix of vegetables when you go food shopping.

18. Choose veggie toppings like spinach, broccoli, and peppers for your pizza.

19. Try eating foods from other countries. Many of these dishes have more vegetables, whole grains, and beans.

20. Buy frozen and low-salt (sodium) canned vegetables if you are on a budget. They may cost less and keep longer than fresh ones.

21. Serve your favorite vegetable and a salad with low-fat macaroni and cheese.

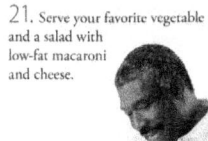

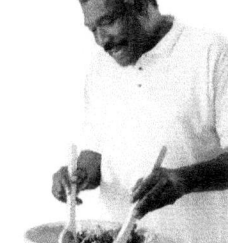

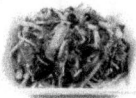

Cook with care, Claire.

22. Stir fry, broil, or bake with non-stick spray or low-salt broth. Cook with less oil and butter.

23. Try not to snack while cooking or cleaning the kitchen.

24. Cook with smaller amounts of cured meats (smoked turkey and turkey bacon). They are high in salt.

Cook in style, Kyle.

25. Cook with a mix of spices instead of salt.

26. Try different recipes for baking or broiling meat, chicken, and fish.

27. Choose foods with little or no added sugar to reduce calories.

28. Choose brown rice instead of white rice.

Eat healthy on the go, Jo.

29. Have a big vegetable salad with low-calorie salad dressing when eating out. Share your main dish with a friend or have the other half wrapped to go.

30. Make healthy choices at fast food restaurants. Try grilled chicken (with skin removed) instead of a cheeseburger.

31. Skip the fries and chips and choose a salad.

32. Order a fruit salad instead of ice cream or cake.

Rethink your drink, Linc.

33. Find a water bottle you really like (from a church or club event, favorite sports team, etc.) and drink water from it every day.

34. Peel and eat an orange instead of drinking orange juice.

35. If you drink whole milk, try changing to 2% milk. It has less fat than whole milk. Once you get used to 2% milk, try 1% or fat-free (skim) milk. This will help you reduce the amount of fat and calories you take in each day.

36. Drink water instead of juice and regular soda.

Eat smart, Bart.

37. Eat foods made from whole grains every day, such as whole wheat bread, brown rice, oats, and whole grain corn.

38. Use whole grain bread for toast and sandwiches.

39. Keep a healthy snack with you, such as fresh fruit, a handful of nuts, and whole grain crackers.

40. Slow down at snack time. Eating a bag of low-fat popcorn takes longer than eating a candy bar.

41. Share a bowl of fruit with family and friends.

42. Eat a healthy snack or meal before shopping for food. Do not shop on an empty stomach.

43. Shop at your local farmers market for fresh, local food.

Keep track, Jack.

44. Make a list of food you need to buy before you go to the store.

45. Keep a written record of what you eat for a week. It can help you see when you tend to overeat or eat foods high in fat or calories.

Read the label, Mabel.

46. Compare food labels on packages.

47. Choose foods lower in saturated fats, trans fats, cholesterol (ko-LESS-tuh-ruhl), calories, salt, and added sugars.

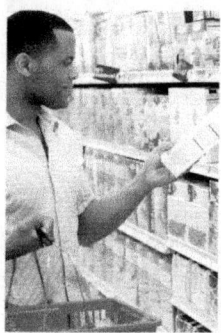

Take Care of Your Mind, Body, and Soul

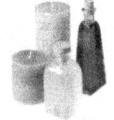
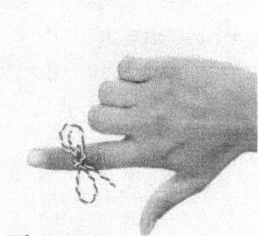

You can exhale, Gail.

48. Take time to change the way you eat and get active. Try one new food or activity a week.

49. Find ways to relax. Try deep breathing, taking a walk, or listening to your favorite music.

50. Pamper yourself. Read a book, take a long bath, or meditate.

51. Think before you eat. Try not to eat when you are bored, upset, or unhappy.

Be Creative

Honor your health as your most precious gift. There are many more ways to prevent or delay type 2 diabetes by making healthy food choices and moving more. Discover your own and share them with your family, friends, and neighbors.

Make up your own, Tyrone or Simone.

52. _____

53. _____

54. _____

Track Your Progress

Visit www.YourDiabetesInfo.org or call 1-888-693-6337 / TTY: 1-866-569-1162 to get your free GAME PLAN to Prevent Type 2 Diabetes booklet. It has charts to help you track the foods you eat and how much you move each day.

Things to Remember:

- Talk to your doctor about your risk for getting type 2 diabetes and what you can do to lower your chances.

- Take steps to prevent diabetes by making healthy food choices, staying at a healthy weight, and moving more every day.

- Find ways to stay calm during your day. Being active and reading a good book can help you lower stress.

- Keep track of the many ways you are moving more and eating healthy by writing them down.

National Diabetes Education Program
1-888-693-NDEP (1-888-693-6337)
www.YourDiabetesInfo.org

Janet O. Brown-Friday, RN, MSN, MPH, Clinical Trials Manager, Diabetes Clinical Trials Unit, Albert Einstein College of Medicine reviewed this material for accuracy.

HHS' NDEP is jointly sponsored by NIH and CDC with the support of more than 200 partner organizations.

By joining a research study, people can help improve their health and the health of others. See www.clinicaltrials.gov and www.cdc.gov/diabetes/projects/index.htm.

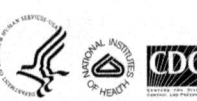

NIH Publication No. 12-5487
NDEP-71
Revised August 2012

The NDEP prints on recycled paper with bio-based ink.

An abundance of materials is available today for anyone wanting to know more about diabetes, dialysis, exercise, and other areas. The National Institute of Health provides a wealth of free information. The Diabetes Education Program is a part of this organization and provides free information as well. These may be obtained by email or phone.

www.ndep.nih.gov
1-800-438-5383

Listed below are just a few of the brochures available free of charge:

THE POWER TO CONTROL DIABETES IS IN YOUR HANDS

*This brochure is designed for older adults to help them manage their diabetes and understand how to check blood sugar levels, manage the ABC's of diabetes, and access Medicare benefits.

HELP A LOVED ONE WITH DIABETES

*This tip sheet provides practical suggestions for helping loved ones with diabetes. It also lists organizations that can help.

FAMILY REUNION HEALTH GUIDE

*A resource to discuss the connection between diabetes, high blood pressure and kidney disease.

As I stood beside the dark granite headstone at Bobby's grave, I could not help but feel as if I wanted to speak directly to him to let him know how I valued this special gift he had given me. The beautifully engraved stone pictured an illustration of a fisherman standing on the bow of a boat, casting a line into the water to fish. A strange feeling came over me as I realized I could have been the person pictured standing in the boat. I suddenly felt a bond or closeness to this person whom I had never met. I assumed that he, too, enjoyed fishing or perhaps time on the water. It seemed we shared a favorite pastime. The background scenery could have been mistaken for the shoreline along our lake where I have enjoyed fishing so many years. To many people, I am sure this image of someone fishing would mean absolutely nothing, but I immediately felt a close connection to this person lying below me, a young man that I never had the opportunity to meet. As my wife strolled over the cemetery, I used the time to be alone with my thoughts as I pondered the changes this young man had made to my life. Finally, I took my pen and wrote a personal message on a card, sealed it in a plastic bag and taped it to the back of the stone so the weather would not destroy it, hoping some member of his family would find it at some time. Several weeks later I received a message from his mother letting me know what my note had meant to her. I was glad we had made the trip to visit Bobby's grave, I felt as if I had found a sort of closure for having done so. If I have been able to convey my feelings about this young man who has done so much to make my life so much better, then I have accomplished a second goal.

Five years have now passed since I received my new pancreas and kidney. Within the last couple of years I had a thorough eye exam and discovered that the lens in my eyes had become cloudy due to years of diabetes and that I had developed something called "sugar cataracts." I underwent lens replacement surgery (commonly known as cataract surgery) and I now have 20/20 vision in one eye and 20/25 vision in the other without glasses. I will continue to require reading glasses. My vision is not quite as good as it was when I was nineteen, but, for someone with a long history of type one diabetes and also sixty-four years old, I am very thankful for my current eyesight today. I am also grateful for the pancreas donated to me which alleviated the daily insulin injections and episodes of hypoglycemia. I am also extremely grateful for the kidney which keeps me from needing dialysis in order to stay alive.

    I also wanted to share some helpful and easily understood information with those currently dealing with diabetes or those seeking to prevent it in the future. By making simple lifestyle changes, many people can avoid becoming a type two diabetic. These changes can be as simple as getting more exercise through walking, or making dietary changes to include a choice of fruits and vegetables. Type two diabetes can often be prevented by simply losing a small amount of weight. These simple changes can often create positive outcomes for many people of varying ages. By including some important and easy to understand diabetic educational materials, I have tried to provide a starting point for those seeking information as they learn about the role diabetes care and prevention can play in their lives.

    Individuals with diabetes today can expect a brighter future based upon the attention paid toward staying healthy and maintaining good blood glucose, blood pressure, and cholesterol levels. It seems the individual with well-controlled diabetes often functions better and has more energy than those with no known medical issues who pay little attention to maintaining a healthy lifestyle. As one doctor told me years ago, "Some of the healthiest patients I have are my diabetic patients. "

    I would also like to encourage everyone to become an organ donor. This could possibly be the greatest gift you will ever make.

Type one diabetic for thirty-five years. . . .

Kidney/ pancreas transplant recipient. . . .
An organ donor. . . .

Sixty-four years' old. . . .

. . . . still having fun!

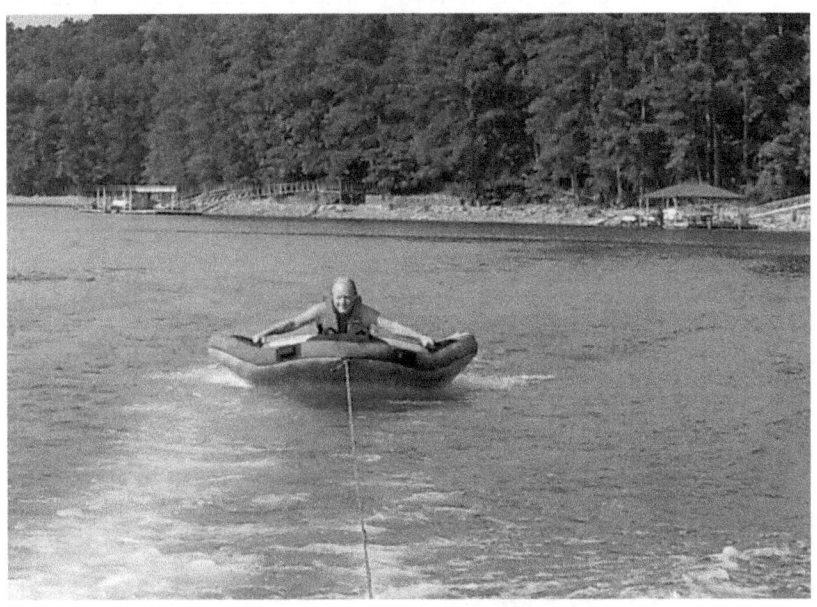

Thanks for reading!

*One of the best sources of information about diabetes can be found in each issue of *diabetic living*. Pages are filled with great information, delicious low-calorie recipes, and other topics to help the person with or without diabetes live a healthier life. Available locally in bookstores and various locations, a digital edition is available on Nook, Kindle Fire, Zinio, and Google Play.

DiabeticLivingOnline.com/digital

To get free recipes and tips sent to your email each week FREE, sign up at:

DiabeticLivingOnline.com/Newsletter

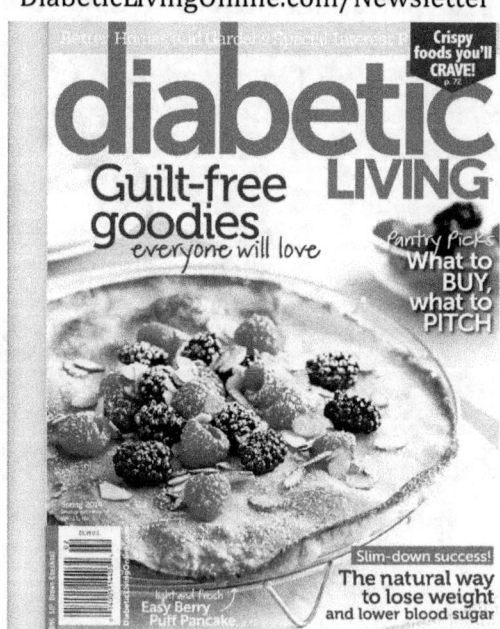

Reference Credits:

Adamec, Christie   2002 The Encyclopedia of Diabetes
    New York, NY: Facts on File, Inc.

Ford-Martin, Paula 2004, The Everything Diabetes Book.
    Avon: F+W Publication Company.

"Diabetes."   World Health Organization International
    Assessed: December 31, 2009

ADDITIONAL RESOURCES

National Diabetes Education Program
1-800-438-5383 or www.ndep.nih.gov and click on the Small Steps logo

American Association of Diabetes Educators
1-800-TEAM-UP4 or www.aadenet.org

American Diabetes Association
1-800-DIABETES or www.diabetes.org

American Dietetic Association
1-800-877-1600 or www.eatright.org

Centers for Disease Control and Prevention
1-877-232-3422 or www.cdc.gov/diabetes

United States Department of Agriculture (USDA)
www.nutrition.gov

Healthier US Initiative
www.healthierus.gov

National Institute of Diabetes and Digestive and Kidney Diseases
National Diabetes Information Clearinghouse
1-800-860-8747 or www.niddk.nih.gov

Weight-Control Information Network
www.win.nih.gov/index.htm

National Heart, Lung, and Blood Institute
301-592-8573 or www.nhlbi.nih.gov

For on-line fat and calorie counters, visit these web sites:

National Heart, Lung, and Blood Institute
http://hp2010.nhlbihin.net/menuplanner/menu.cgi

United States Department of Agriculture
Nutrient Data Laboratory
www.nal.usda.gov/fnic/foodcomp/search/

Acknowledgments

Mrs. Virginia Morton

A great mother-in-law, you convinced me to share my story. I wish you could have been here to read the book.

Mrs. Susan Henderson

A true friend and colleague many years, I cannot thank you enough for your assistance toward the completion of this book. Your editing skills and suggestions were invaluable.